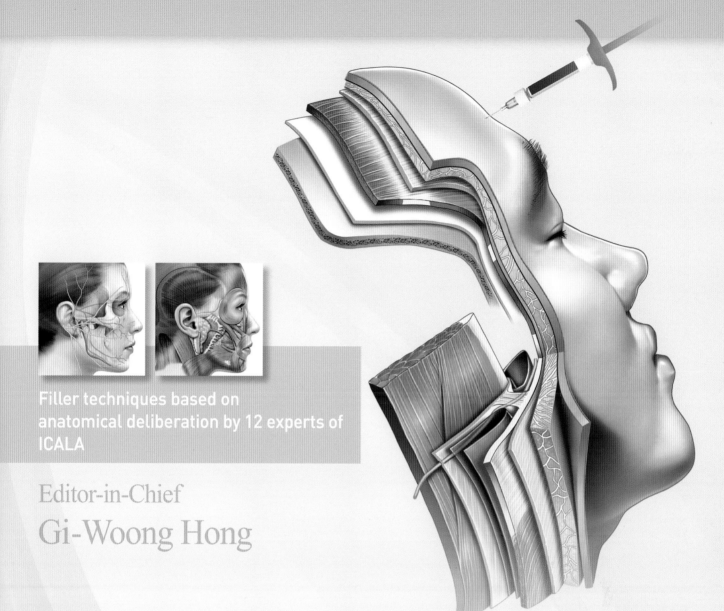

Filler techniques based on anatomical deliberation by 12 experts of ICALA

Editor-in-Chief
Gi-Woong Hong

Practical Guidelines for
Effective and
Safe Filler Injections

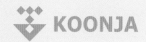 KOONJA

Practical Guidelines for
Effective and Safe Filler Injections

Filler techniques based on anatomical anatomical deliberation by 12 experts of ICALA

First edition printed | February 27, 2019
First edition published | March 14, 2019

Written by   Gi-Woong Hong, 11 others
Published by   Ju-yeon Jang
Planned by   Sung-jae Lee
Edited by   Mi-ae Park
Editing Design by   Eun-mi Joo
Cover Design by   Jae-wook Kim
Illustrations by   Ho-hyeon Lee
Produced by   Sang-hyeon Shin
Publishing House   Koonja Publishing Company
                    Registration No. 4-139 (June 24, 1991)
                    Paju Publishing Complex, 338, Hoedong-gil (474-1 Seopae-dong),
                    Paju-si, Gyeonggi-do, South Korea (10881)
                    Telephone : (031) 943-1888   Fax : (031) 955-9545
                    Website : www.koonja.co.kr

ISBN   979-11-5955-417-9

Practical Guidelines for
Effective and
Safe Filler Injections

Authors

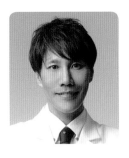

Gi-Woong Hong, M.D., Ph.D., Plastic Surgeon

Director of SAMSKIN Plastic Surgery Clinic
Clinical Professor of Department of Plastic Surgery, Chung-Ang University Medical Center
Member of the Korean Society of Plastic and Reconstructive Surgeon
Member of the Korean Society of Aesthetic Plastic Surgery
Scientific Committee of Korean Association of Minimal Invasive Plastic Surgery (MIPS)
President of International Clinical Aesthetic Leaders Academy (ICALA)

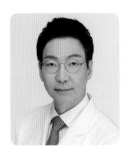

Ee-Seok Lim, M.D., Ph.D., Dermatologist

Director of Lim Ee-Seok Thema Dermatologic Clinic
Chairman of Korean Academy of Corrective Dermatology
Chairman of Korean Society Hair Restoration Treatment
Chairman of Korean Clinical Skin Surgery Research Society
Chairman of Dermatologist Forum for Cosmetic Research and Education
President of International Clinical Aesthetic Leaders Academy (ICALA)

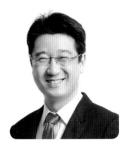

Won Lee, M.D., Ph.D., Plastic Surgeon, English version editor

Director of Yonsei E1 Plastic Surgery Clinic
Outclinic Professor of the Department of Plastic Surgery of CHA Medical Center
Member of the Korean Society of Plastic and Reconstructive Surgeons & APS
Scientific Committee of Korean Association of Minimal Invasive Plastic Surgery (MIPS)
Committee of International Clinical Aesthetic Leaders Academy (ICALA)

Choon-Shik Youn, M.D., Dermatologist

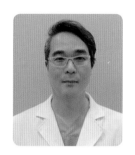

Director of Yemiwon Dermatologic Clinic
Advisory Board Member of Department of Dermatology, Seoul National University Hospital
General Secretary of Korean Society for Anti-Aging Dermatology
Academic Committee of the Association of Korean Dermatologist
Member of Korean Dermatological Association
Committee of International Clinical Aesthetic Leaders Academy (ICALA)

Dae-Hyun Kim, M.D., Dermatologist

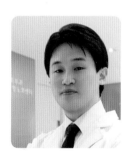

Director of Widwin Dermatologic Clinic
Assistant Administrator of the Association of Korean Dermatologists
Assistant Administrator of Korean Society for Anti-Aging Dermatology
Member of Korean Dermatological Association
Committee of International Clinical Aesthetic Leaders Academy (ICALA)

Eui-Sik Kim, M.D., Ph.D., Plastic Surgeon

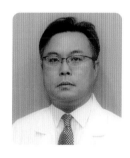

Director of Friends Plastic Surgery Clinic
Visiting Professor of Department of Plastic Surgery, Chonnam National University Medical School
Scientific Committee of Korean Association of Minimal Invasive Plastic Surgery (MIPS)
Member of the Korean Society of Plastic and Reconstructive Surgeon
Member of the Korean Society of Aesthetic Plastic Surgery
Committee of International Clinical Aesthetic Leaders Academy (ICALA)

Authors

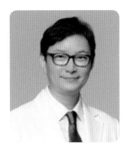

Hyung-Ik Baik, M.D., Plastic Surgeon

Director of BYUL Plastic Surgery Clinic
Member of the Korean Society of Plastic and Reconstructive Surgeon
Member of the Korean Society of Aesthetic Plastic Surgery
Scientific Committee of Korean Association of Minimal Invasive Plastic Surgery (MIPS)
Committee of International Clinical Aesthetic Leaders Academy (ICALA)

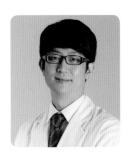

Hyun-Jo Kim, M.D., M.S., Dermatologist

Director of CNP Skin Clinic, Cheonan & Director of CNP Holdings
Visiting Professor of Department of Dermatology, Soonchunhyang University College of Medicine
Director of Korean Society of Anti-Aging Dermatology
Scholarship Assistant Administrator of the Association of Korean Dermatologists
3rd & 4th Annual Congress Chairman of Global Association of Leaders in Aesthetics and Anatomy
Committee of International Clinical Aesthetic Leaders Academy (ICALA)

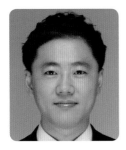

Jeong-Jun Park, M.D., Ph.D., Plastic Surgeon

Director of Dream Up Plastic surgery clinic
Member of the Korean Society of Plastic and Reconstructive Surgeons
Member of the Korean Society of Aesthetic Plastic Surgery
Member of International Confederation of Plastic, Reconstructive and Aesthetic Surgery
Committee of International Clinical Aesthetic Leaders Academy (ICALA)

Yong-Woo Lee, M.D., M.B.A., Plastic Surgeon

Director of LIKE Plastic Surgery Clinic
Member of the Korean Society of Plastic and Reconstructive Surgeon
Member of the Korean Society of Aesthetic Plastic Surgery
Scientific Committee of Korean Association of Minimal Invasive Plastic Surgery (MIPS)
Committee of International Clinical Aesthetic Leaders Academy (ICALA)

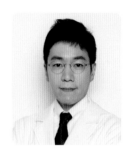

Yu-Ri Kim, M.D., Ph.D., Dermatologist

Director of Chois Dermatologic Clinic
Member of Korean Dermatological Association
Member of Korean Society for Aesthetic and Dermatologic Surgery
Committee of International Clinical Aesthetic Leaders Academy (ICALA)

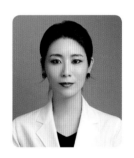

Won-Sug Jung, M.D., Ph.D., Anatomist

Assistant professor, Dept. of Anatomy, Gachon University School of Medicine
Graduate course in Yonsei University, Korea, Ph.D. degree
Yonsei University, College of Medicine, Korea, Medical Doctor

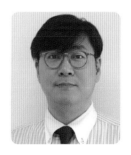

Authors

Soft tissue filler injection is one of the most commonly performed cosmetic procedures that has greatly progressed in the last 10 years.

However, with progress, there are no precise guidelines; rather, when administering filler injections, following the previous guidelines may result in the selection of the wrong procedures.

The purpose of this book was to (1) identify the correct procedure in various approaching methods and (2) show the progress in identifying the correct method of filler injection.

The authors tried to identify the correct method based on anatomy. Precise anatomical knowledge would lead to efficient and safe injection guidelines.

The components of this book are as follows; anatomist professor's description about the precise anatomy for filler injection, plastic surgery specialist and dermatology specialist's description of their techniques, and an organized table at the end of each chapter. In this book, various experienced opinions by specialist physicians of anatomy, plastic surgery, and dermatology and several ideas when actually administering injections are reported.

Each technique may follow the same or different method, suggesting that there are no formulated filler injection techniques. On reading this book, every physician will compare the techniques described to their own and will perform the technique better with better results.

This is still insufficient to cover all procedure but we hope to help improve the preciseness and safety of filler techniques.

International Clinical Aesthetic Leaders Academy (ICALA)

Contents

Contents

Contents

Chapter **13** **Infraorbital hollowness** 243

Chapter **14** **Pretarsal fullness** 291

Anatomy

Won-Sug Jung, M.D., Ph.D., Anatomist

CHAPTER 01 Anatomy

1. 1 Layers of the face

The face basically consists of 5 layers, namely, skin, subcutaneous layers, superficial musculoaponeurotic system (SMAS), loose areolar tissues, and deep fascia (Fig. 1-1).

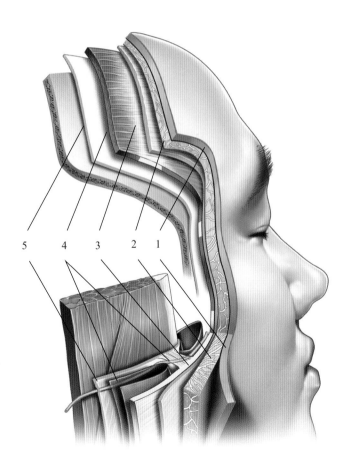

1. Skin
2. Subcutaneous layer
3. Superficial musculo-aponeurotic system
4. Retaining ligaments and spaces
5. Periosteum and deep fascia

Fig. 1-1 Layers of the face

1. 1. 1 Skin

The thickness of the skin varies between the regions. The skin of the eyelids is the thinnest, while that of the cheek and nasal tip is the thickest. However, there are some literatures reporting that the neck area is the thickest.

1. 1. 2 Subcutaneous layer

This is also known as superficial fat and is divided into multiple compartments (Fig. 1-2). Superficial fat ptosis occurs during the aging process.

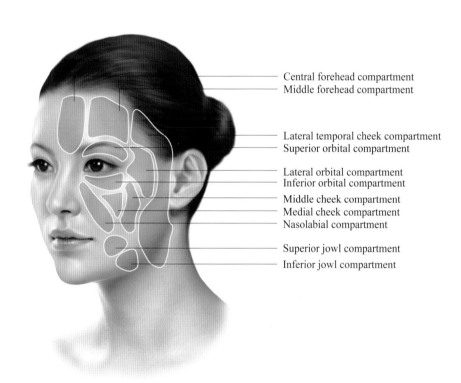

Central forehead compartment
Middle forehead compartment

Lateral temporal cheek compartment
Superior orbital compartment

Lateral orbital compartment
Inferior orbital compartment
Middle cheek compartment
Medial cheek compartment
Nasolabial compartment

Superior jowl compartment
Inferior jowl compartment

Fig. 1-2 Superficial fat compartments

1. 1. 3 SMAS (Superficial Musculo-aponeurotic System)

Mimetic muscles and related SMAS will be discussed in the section on muscles of the face (Chapter 1.3).

1. 1. 4 Loose areolar tissues

Multiple named spaces, retaining ligaments, and deep fat compartments are located in this layer. Facial nerves are located deeper than the SMAS. The prezygomatic, premaxillary, premasseteric, and deep piriform spaces are located in this layer (Fig. 1-3). Retaining ligaments are classified as true (attached to bone) and false (attached muscle fascia) ligaments and are attached to the dermal layer to reinforce the boundaries of spaces (Fig. 1-4). Deep fat compartments consist of suborbicularis oculi fat (SOOF), retroorbicularis oculi fat (ROOF), deep medial cheek fat, and buccal fat pads; the volume of decreases during the aging process.

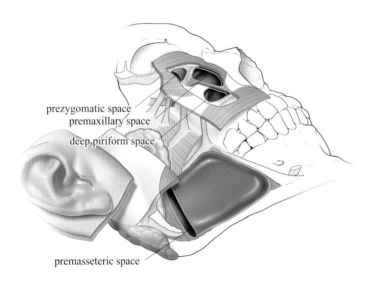

Fig. 1-3 **Facial spaces**

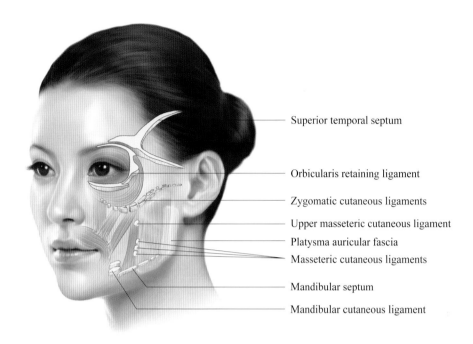

Fig. 1-4 **Retaining ligaments of the face**

Labels:
- Superior temporal septum
- Orbicularis retaining ligament
- Zygomatic cutaneous ligaments
- Upper masseteric cutaneous ligament
- Platysma auricular fascia
- Masseteric cutaneous ligaments
- Mandibular septum
- Mandibular cutaneous ligament

1. 1. 5 Deep fascia and periosteum

The deep fascia is the continuing structure from the periosteum, which covers the temporalis and masseter muscles. The deep temporal fascia (DTF) is divided into the deep and superficial layer and attached to the upper border of the zygomatic arch. The parotido-masseteric fascia continues to the mandibular periosteum and covers the masseter muscle and parotid gland and also attaches to the zygomatic arch.

1. 1. 6 Skull

Asian skulls are different from Western skulls, in which the front-occipital length is shorter and horizontal width is larger. The height is also taller. It also has a more prominent zygoma, more depressed nasal bone, and shorter nasal spine. Bone resorption changes with the aging process, and volume decreases at the infraorbital area, but there are no known changes at the orbit and piriform aperture compared to the Western skull (Fig. 1-5).

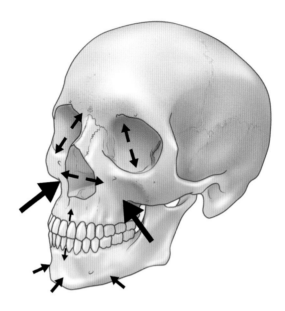

Fig. 1-5 **Bone change with aging**

1. 2 **Muscles of the face**

The first group is the mastication muscles from the first pharyngeal arch, and the second group is the facial expression muscles (mimetic muscles) from the second pharyngeal arch. Facial expression muscles are innervated by the facial nerve and are located at the third layer, connected with the galea aponeurotica, superficial temporal fascia (STF), and SMAS. These muscles are attached to the skin and form wrinkles when constricted, and these wrinkles are perpendicular to the muscle fiber direction (Fig. 1-6, 1-7).

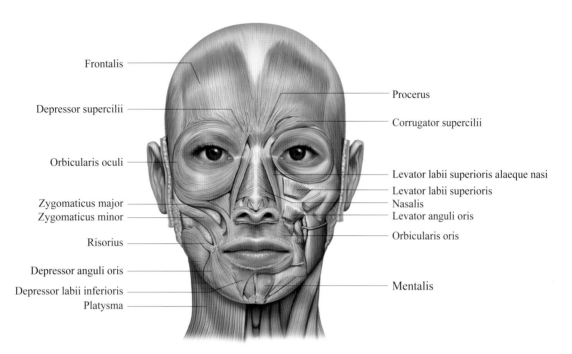

Fig. 1-6 Muscles of facial expression: Anterior view

Frontalis

Depressor supercilii

Orbicularis oculi

Zygomaticus major
Zygomaticus minor

Risorius

Depressor anguli oris

Depressor labii inferioris
Platysma

Procerus

Corrugator supercilii

Levator labii superioris alaeque nasi
Levator labii superioris
Nasalis
Levator anguli oris

Orbicularis oris

Mentalis

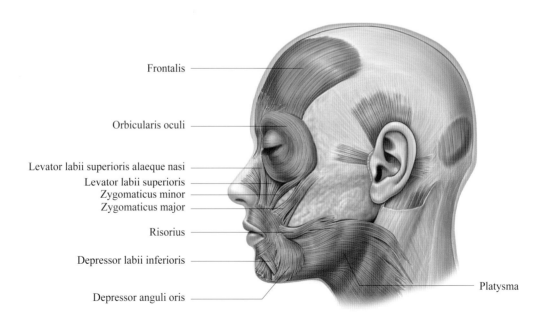

Fig. 1-7 Muscles of facial expression: Lateral view

Frontalis

Orbicularis oculi

Levator labii superioris alaeque nasi
Levator labii superioris
Zygomaticus minor
Zygomaticus major

Risorius

Depressor labii inferioris

Depressor anguli oris

Platysma

1. 2. 1 Muscles of the upper face

1. 2. 1. 1 Frontalis muscle

The frontalis muscle is a part of the occipitofrontalis muscle and originates from the galea aponeurotica and runs inferiorly and attaches to the orbicularis oculi, procerus, depressor supercilii, and corrugator supercilii muscles. Thus, there are no attachments between the frontalis muscle and skull, and the galeal fat pad is located between them.

The frontalis muscle is rectangular in shape and consists of two bellies bilaterally. They fuse together at the lower part of the forehead but divide bilaterally at the average level of 47 mm above the supraorbital margin. The heights of bifurcation are variable, and in 10% of the population, they are not divided. The frontalis muscle is the only muscle responsible for raising the eyebrows and forming horizontal wrinkle of the forehead, and different shapes of wrinkles reflect different frontalis muscle formations. The lateral end of the frontalis muscle is located at an average level of 9 mm lateral to the temporal crest.

1. 2. 1. 2 Procerus muscle

Procerus muscle is an inverted triangular shape small muscle that originates from the nasal bone and lateral nasal cartilage and runs in a trapezoidal shape to attach to the glabella area skin interconnecting the frontalis muscle. It forms nasal horizontal wrinkles by pulling the glabella.

1. 2. 1. 3 Depressor supercilii muscle

The depressor supercilii muscle originates from the frontal process of the maxilla just below the frontomaxillary suture and runs upward and attaches to the medial eyebrow skin, which is located 15mm above the medial palpebral ligament. It functions in tandem with the corrugator supercilii muscle in pulling the medial eyebrow downward.

1. 2. 1. 4 Corrugator supercilii muscle

The corrugator supercilii muscle is covered by the orbicularis oculi muscle and located deeper. It originates from the medial end of the superciliary arch bony part and runs in superior lateral direction and is interconnected with the frontalis muscle and attached to the middle of the supraorbital margin skin. Thus, it is located deeply at the origin site but superficially at the end. The widths are 1cm at origin and 2 cm at the eyebrow portion, and the lateral part is located A point(15 mm, 15 mm) to B point(35 mm, 30 mm) from the medial canthus. It forms the glabellar perpendicular wrinkle by pulling the medial eyebrow medially and downward.

1. 2. 2 Muscles of the midface

1. 2. 2. 1 Orbicularis oculi muscle

Its function is to close the eye surrounded by the palpebral fissure and works as a sphincter. The lateral part is larger, so the muscle looks like aviator's sunglasses. It is divided into the orbital part from the bone and palpebral part from the medial palpebral ligament, and the palpebral part is divided again into the preseptal and pretarsal parts. The palpebral part works to close the eyes softly, and the orbital part works to close the eyes tightly, forming the crow's feet. The lateral part of the orbicularis oculi runs vertically, so it works against the frontalis muscle and pulls the lateral eyebrow downward.

The orbital part muscle fibers are mostly round in shape, but there are two portions that are not continuous and exist as muscle bundles. In the lateral part, there is a lateral band, and in the medial part, there is a medial band. The outer margin of the orbicularis oculi is located at the point 4:6 when we draw a line from the lateral canthus to the tragus and located 1cm laterally from the frontal process of the zygomatic bone.

1. 2. 2. 2 Nasalis muscle

It consists of the upper transverse and lower alar parts. The transverse part originates from the maxilla and runs in superior medial direction and attaches to the SMAS with opposite transverse muscle fibers. The alar part originates from the maxilla just above the lateral incisor and canine and inserts to the deep skin layer of the lower lateral cartilage (major alar cartilage) lateral crus. When the lateral part constricts, it compresses the nostril, so it is also called as the compressor naris, and when the alar part constricts, it dilates the nostril, so it is also called as the dilator naris.

1. 2. 2. 3 Depressor septi nasi muscle

It originates from the maxilla just above the central incisor and anterior nasal spine, runs in the columella, and attaches to the lower lateral cartilage medial crus. It helps to dilate the nostril by pulling the nasal tip.

1. 2. 2. 4 Levator labii superioris alaeque nasi muscle

It originates from the frontal process of the maxilla and divides into two fibers, and the medial part attaches to the alar, and the lateral part attaches to the upper lip skin and nasolabial fold. It dilates the nostril and pulls the upper lip upward.

1. 2. 2. 5 Levator labii superioris muscle

It originates 1cm below the infraorbital margin and above the infraorbital foramen and is covered by the orbicularis oculi muscle. It runs downward and attaches to the upper lip skin and alar. It is located between the levator labii superioris alaeque nasi muscle and zygomaticus minor muscle and deeper than these two muscles.

1. 2. 2. 6 Zygomaticus minor muscle

It originates from the zygomatic bone combined with the orbicularis oculi muscle and runs downward and attaches to the upper lip skin and alar. Its running direction is very variable such as the oblique or horizontal direction and falls downward abruptly.

The origins of the levator labii superioris alaeque nasi muscle, levator labii superioris muscle, and zygomaticus minor muscle are widely separated, but when running downward, they gather and attach to the orbicularis oris muscle surface to pull the upper lip upward. Moreover, they have fibers attaching to the alar.

1. 2. 2. 7 Levator anguli oris muscle

It is located deep and covered by levator labii superioris muscle and originates from the canine fossa, lower than the infraorbital foramen, and attaches the modiolus to other muscles.

1. 2. 2. 8 Zygomaticus major muscle

It originates near the zygomaticomaxillary suture and runs downward to attach to the modiolus. It is divided into two or three bellies, and some attach to the skin to form a cheek dimple. The levator anguli oris muscle runs downward between the superficial and deep bellies of the zygomaticus major muscle.

1. 2. 2. 9 Orbicularis oris muscle

It is rather a sphincter muscle around the oral fissure than two bellies of muscle connecting at the bilateral modiolus. It can be divided into the marginal and peripheral parts by the vermilion border. When constricted, the lips can be pouted anteriorly. It forms the smoker's line when the aging process proceeds.

1. 2. 2. 10 Buccinator muscle

It originates from the maxillary and mandibular alveolar processes and pterygomandibular raphe and combines with the orbicularis oris muscle and attaches to the modiolus. The upper and lower bands proceed anteriorly, but the middle bands on the upper and lower parts decussate each other. The parotid duct perforates the buccinator muscle. When chewing, the cheeks are compressed to the teeth, not having space between the teeth and cheek so that food cannot be stagnated. Moreover, the buccinator muscle acts when blowing hard.

1. 2. 2. 11 Risorius muscle

It is located superficially and runs horizontally and attaches to the modiolus, but the fiber shapes and directions are very variable. Usually, it covers the anterior part of the masseter muscle. It pulls the mouth corner laterally when smiling.

1. 2. 3 Muscles of the lower face

1. 2. 3. 1 Depressor anguli oris muscle

It is located superficially and originates from the wide area of the mandible, lateral from the mental tubercle, and runs upward and becomes narrow to attach to the modiolus. Some fibers transform to the transversus menti at the mental tubercle. The depressor anguli muscle is triangular in shape and has a concave muscle border. When drawing the vertical line of the modiolus, the anterior border is located 30° anteriorly, and the posterior border is located 45° posteriorly. It pulls the mouth corner downward when presenting a sad expression.

1. 2. 3. 2 Depressor labii inferioris muscle

It is located deeper than the depressor anguli oris muscle and runs in superior medial direction and attaches to the lower lip skin and mucosa.

1. 2. 3. 3 Platysma muscle

It is a wide, thin, and flat muscle and originates from the muscle fascia of the pectoralis major and deltoid muscles. It runs across the clavicle and in superior medial direction. Sometimes, medial border fibers are decussated at the midline of the mentum. It attaches to the lower border of mandible and sometimes runs deeper than the depressor anguli oris and risorius muscles and attaches at the level of the zygomatic arch. When contracted muscle bundles are seen at the neck skin, the mouth corner is pulled downward when showing a sad expression. When elasticity decreases due to the aging process, gobbler neck deformity could develop at the prominent medial border of the platysma.

1. 2. 3. 4 Mentalis muscle

It is a cone-shaped muscle that originates from the anterior mandible incisive fossa and runs downward to attach to the mentum skin. When contracted mentum skin is pulled upward, the lower lip pouts anteriorly, and a walnut appearance is shown at the mentum skin.

1. 2. 4 Muscles of mastication

It originates from first pharyngeal arch and starts from skull and attaches to the mandible. Its main action is chewing. It is innervated by the mandibular branch of the trigeminal nerve and covered by the deep fascia, which is the continuation of the periosteum. The lateral and medial pterygoid muscles are located deeper than the mandible, so it will omit about two muscles (Fig. 1-8).

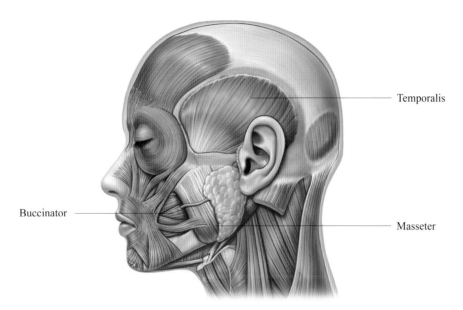

Fig. 1-8 Muscles of mastication

1. 2. 4. 1 Temporalis muscle

It is located at the temporal fossa and originates widely from the skull below the inferior temporal line and becomes narrow as it runs downward. It transverses inside the zygomatic arch and attaches to the inner side of the coronoid process of the mandible. The temporalis muscle is the most potent elevator of the mandible, and muscle fibers are fan shaped, and posterior muscle fibers pull the mandible in the posterior direction. The deep temporal fat pad (DTFP) (temporal lobe of the buccal fat pad), which is an extension of the buccal fat pad, is located between the temporalis muscle and DTF near the zygomatic arch area.

1. 2. 4. 2 Masseter muscle

It originates from the zygomatic bone and arch and attaches to the mandibular border widely. It divides into three layers. The superficial layer is the largest and originates from the maxillary process of the zygomatic bone and anterior 2/3 of the zygomatic arch and attaches to the mandibular angle border. The middle layer originates from the anterior 2/3 of the zygomatic arch inner border and posterior

1/3 of the zygomatic arch lower border and attaches to the middle of the mandible. The deep layer originates from the zygomatic deep portion and attaches to the upper mandible. It is potent elevator of the mandible.

1. 3 Facial vessels

There are external and internal carotid artery branches at the face. The external carotid artery branches are the facial and superficial temporal arteries. The internal carotid artery branch is the ophthalmic artery. Moreover, the ophthalmic artery branches are the supraorbital, supratrochlear, and dorsal nasal arteries (Fig. 1-9).

The facial artery is branched from the external carotid artery and runs inside the mandible. It circumflexes the mandibular border at the level of the anterior border of the masseter muscle and runs in a

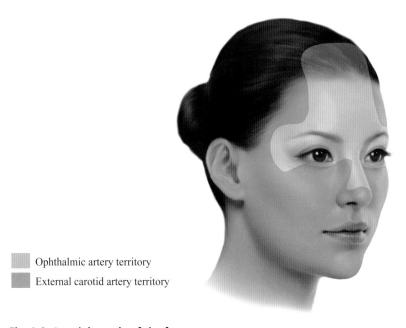

⬜ Ophthalmic artery territory
⬛ External carotid artery territory

Fig. 1-9 Arterial supply of the face

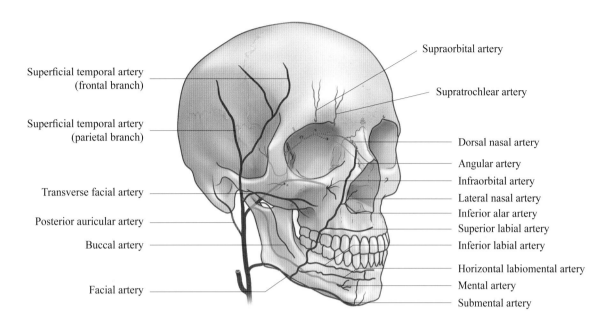

Superficial temporal artery (frontal branch)

Superficial temporal artery (parietal branch)

Transverse facial artery

Posterior auricular artery

Buccal artery

Facial artery

Supraorbital artery

Supratrochlear artery

Dorsal nasal artery

Angular artery

Infraorbital artery

Lateral nasal artery

Inferior alar artery

Superior labial artery

Inferior labial artery

Horizontal labiomental artery

Mental artery

Submental artery

Fig. 1-10 Arterial branches of the face

zigzag pattern in the medial canthus direction. It branches into the inferior labial, superior labial, inferior alar, and lateral nasal and angular arteries. However, these branches vary between populations. Of the Korean population, 36% have all branches described before, and 44% stop until the lateral nasal artery branches. Moreover, only 50% have bilaterally symmetrical arterial distribution in the face (Fig. 1-10).

In 30%, the facial artery does not run in the traditional superior medial direction but runs vertically at the level of mouth corner to the lower border of orbicularis oculi muscle. It is located superficially at the zygomaticus major and risorius muscles and runs tortuously. It runs 5mm from nasolabial fold in 40% and across the nasolabial fold in 1/3.

At the glabella and nose, ophthalmic artery branches such as the supraorbital, supratrochlear, and dorsal nasal arteries are located and form an anastomosis with the external carotid artery branches.

The superficial temporal artery is divided into the parietal and frontal branches and located at the temple and lateral forehead. The frontal branch forms an anastomosis with the ophthalmic artery branches.

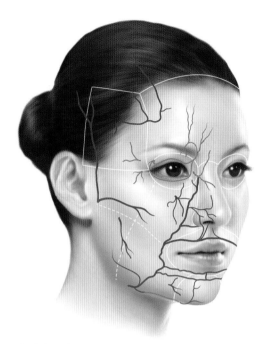

Fig. 1-11 Arteries supplying facial regions

Sometimes, it branches into the transverse facial and zygomatico-orbital arteries.

Furthermore, maxillary artery branches from the external carotid artery perforate the skull and are distributed to the face as the infraorbital, buccal, and mental arteries (Fig. 1-11).

1. 3. 1 Perioral arteries

The facial artery branches into the horizontal labiomental artery between the cheilion and lower border of the mandible. The horizontal labiomental artery runs horizontally along the labiomental crease. Sometimes, it branches into the vertical labiomental artery, forming an anastomosis with the inferior labial and/or mental artery.

The inferior labial artery is branched from the facial artery at the level of the mouth corner height and runs along the vermilion border. In approximately 50%, only the horizontal labiomental artery exists without the inferior labial artery.

The inferior labial artery runs deeper than the orbicularis oris muscle, near the oral mucosa, and tends to run superficially to the skin at the medial side.

The superior labial artery is branched from the facial artery at 1 cm superolateral distance from the mouth corner. It runs horizontally 0.5~1.2 cm from the upper lip vermilion border.

It runs near the oral mucosa which is deeper than the orbicularis oris muscle and branches into the nasal septal artery at the philtrum. The nasal septal artery has one branch that runs deeper into the orbicularis oris muscle and another branch that runs superficial to the muscle. The superficial branch becomes the columellar artery.

At 10%, the inferior alar artery and lateral nasal arteries are branched from the superior labial artery.

1. 3. 2 Perinasal arteries

The inferior alar artery runs to the alar base, and the lateral nasal artery runs to the nasal tip.

The dorsal nasal artery from the ophthalmic artery branch is located at the nasal root, and the anterior ethmoidal artery external nasal branch perforates the rhinion.

The dorsal nasal artery runs between the fibromuscular and deep fatty layers.

At 20%, the dorsal nasal artery and lateral nasal arteries run to the contralateral side crossing the midline.

1. 3. 3 Periocular arteries

The angular artery is the end of the facial artery at 50%. At 25%, it branches from the ophthalmic artery, and at 25%, it does not exist. As mentioned before, 30% of the facial artery runs vertically from the mouth corner and along the border of the orbicularis oculi muscle and directs to the medial canthus, so the angular artery location has many variations.

The eyelids are supplied by the medial palpebral artery from the supratrochlear and lateral palpebral arteries from the lacrimal artery. The lower medial palpebral artery runs deeper than the orbicularis oculi muscle palpebral part.

1. 3. 4 Glabella and forehead arteries

The supratrochlear artery is located at the glabella and central forehead. It exits the orbit and perforates the orbicularis oculi muscle at the level of the medial canthal vertical line and runs superficially. Fifty percent of the supratrochlear artery runs along the glabella frown line.

The supraorbital artery perforates the supraorbital notch/foramen and runs deeper than the orbicularis oculi and frontalis muscles and perforates the frontalis muscle 3 cm lateral from the medial canthus and 2cm above the orbital rim. It forms an anastomosis with the supratrochlear artery medially and superficial temporal artery laterally.

1. 3. 5 Temple arteries

The superficial temporal artery perforates the parotid gland and divides the parietal and frontal branches 18 mm anteriorly and 37 mm superiorly from the tragus. The frontal branch runs in superior medial direction covered by the STF and superficial than the frontalis muscle with connecting supratrochlear artery.

The zygomatico-orbital artery is branched from the superficial temporal artery and runs to the lateral canthus.

The zygomaticotemporal artery is branched from the lacrimal artery and supplies the anterior temple area.

The middle temporal and deep temporal arteries supply the temporalis muscle.

1. 3. 6 Cheek area arteries

The transverse facial artery is branched from the superficial temporal artery inside the parotid glands and runs 1.5cm from the zygomatic arch and supplies the superior lateral cheek.

The buccal artery from the maxillary artery and zygomaticofacial artery from the lacrimal artery supply the inferior medial cheek.

1. 3. 7 Venous supply of the face

The vein location is similar to the arterial location, but there are some exceptions such as those in the inferior ophthalmic and retromandibular veins. The facial vein runs straightly compared to the tortuous facial artery and located 1.5cm posterior to the facial artery. The facial vein runs into the internal jugu-

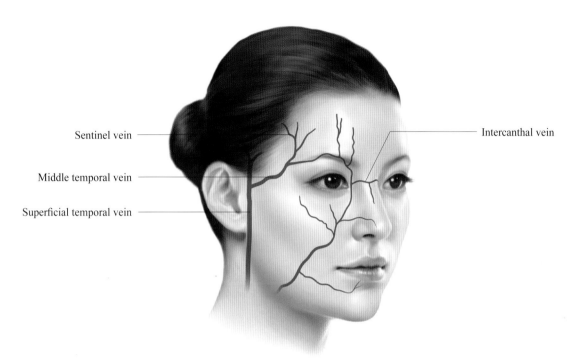

Sentinel vein

Middle temporal vein

Superficial temporal vein

Intercanthal vein

Fig. 1-12 Veins of the face

lar vein but can also run to the ophthalmic vein and into the cavernous sinus.

The intercanthal vein that communicates with the bilateral angular vein exists in 70%.

At the temple area, the middle temporal vein is located 2cm above he zygomatic arch between the superficial and deep layers of the DTF. This vein flows to the superficial temporal vein and communicates with the cavernous sinus through the periocular and superior ophthalmic veins (Fig. 1-12).

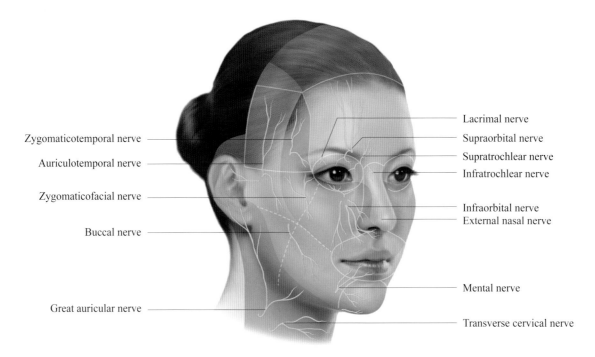

Lacrimal nerve
Supraorbital nerve
Supratrochlear nerve
Infratrochlear nerve

Zygomaticotemporal nerve

Auriculotemporal nerve

Zygomaticofacial nerve

Infraorbital nerve
External nasal nerve

Buccal nerve

Mental nerve

Great auricular nerve

Transverse cervical nerve

Fig. 1-13 **Sensory innervation of the face**

1. 4 Nerves of the face

Sensory innervation of the face and neck are the trigeminal nerve and cervical plexus branches. Facial expression muscles are innervated by the facial nerve branches, and mastication muscles are innervated by the mandibular nerve.

Trigeminal nerve branches usually perforate the skull foramen and innervate the facial skin, and cervical plexus branches innervate the lateral and lower parts of the cheek, part of the ear, and anterior neck skin (Fig. 1-13). The facial nerve divides into five branches in the parotid gland and is covered by SMAS and innervates the deep part of facial expression muscles.

1. 4. 1 Ophthalmic nerve (CNV1)

It is the upper trunk of the trigeminal nerve and penetrates the orbit by the superior orbital fissure and divides into the frontal, nasociliary, and lacrimal nerve. The frontal nerve divides into the supraorbital and supratrochlear nerves, the nasociliary nerve divides into the infratrochlear and external nasal nerves and innervates the forehead, scalp, glabella, eyelid, and nose.

1. 4. 2 Maxillary nerve (CNV2)

It is the middle trunk of the trigeminal nerve and branches into the zygomatic nerve. It terminates to become the infraorbital nerve. The infraorbital nerve widely innervates the lower eyelid, lateral part of the nose, and upper lip. The zygomatic nerve perforates the zygomatic foramen and branches into the zygomaticofacial and zygomaticotemporal nerves (ZTNs).

1. 4. 3 Mandibular nerve (CNV3)

It is the lower trunk of the trigeminal nerve and branches into the motor nerve of the mastication muscle and sensory nerves of the facial skin and head.

The auriculotemporal nerve runs across the parotid gland and in the anterosuperior ear direction and innervates the anterior ear and temple area. The buccal nerve perforates the buccinator muscle and innervates part of the cheek. The mental nerve perforates the mental foramen and innervates the lower lip and chin.

1. 4. 4 Cervical plexus

The cervical plexus emerges at the middle posterior border of the sternocleidomastoid muscle. The great auricular nerve innervates the mastoid process, parotid gland region, and mandibular angle skin, and the transverse cervical nerve innervates the anterior triangle of neck skin.

1. 4. 5 Facial nerve (Fig. 1-14)

The temporal branch consists of multiple branches. After perforating the parotid gland, it crosses the zygomatic arch and innervates the frontalis muscle, corrugator supercilii muscle, and upper part of the

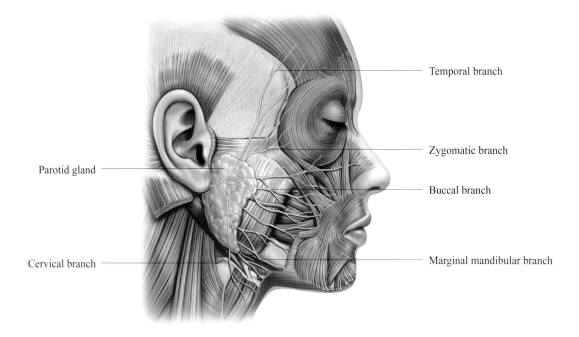

Temporal branch

Zygomatic branch

Parotid gland

Buccal branch

Cervical branch

Marginal mandibular branch

Fig. 1-14 **Facial nerve**

orbicularis oculi muscle.

The zygomatic branch innervates the lower part of the orbicularis oculi, zygomaticus major, and zygomaticus minor muscles.

The buccal branch runs along the parotid duct and innervates the elevator muscles of the upper lip.

The zygomatic and buccal branches join together and innervate the nasalis, procerus, and corrugator supercilii muscles.

The marginal mandibular branch innervates the lower part of the orbicularis oris, depressor anguli oris, depressor labii inferioris, and mentalis muscles.

The cervical branch innervates the platysma muscle.

02

Cadaveric anatomy

02 Cadaveric anatomy

ICALA

2. 1 Layers of the face

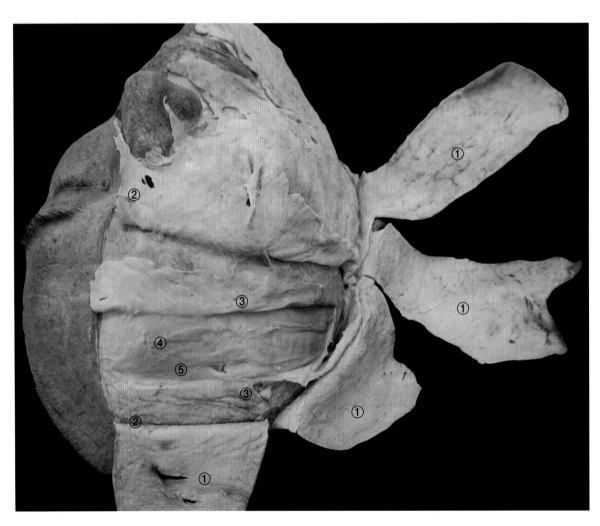

Fig. 2-1 Layers of the face ① Skin ② Subcutaneous layer(=superficial fatty layer) ③ SMAS ④ Loose areolar tissues ⑤ Periosteum

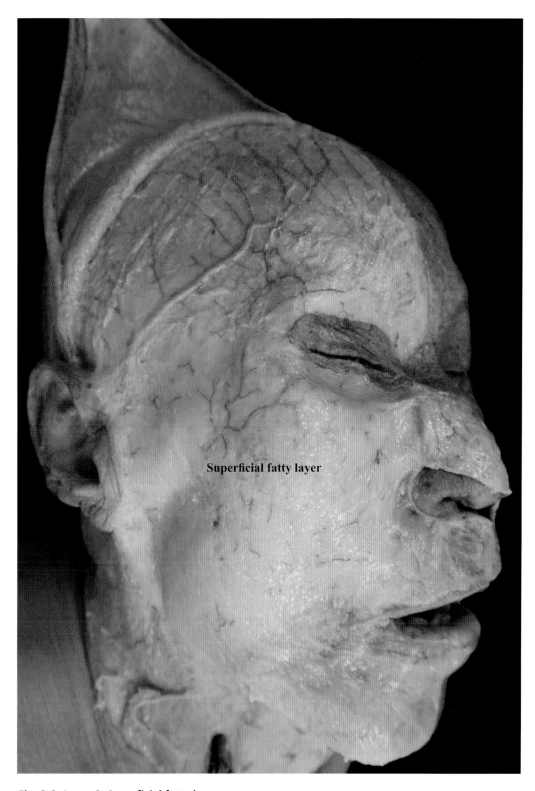

Fig. 2-2 **Layer 2; Superficial fatty layer**

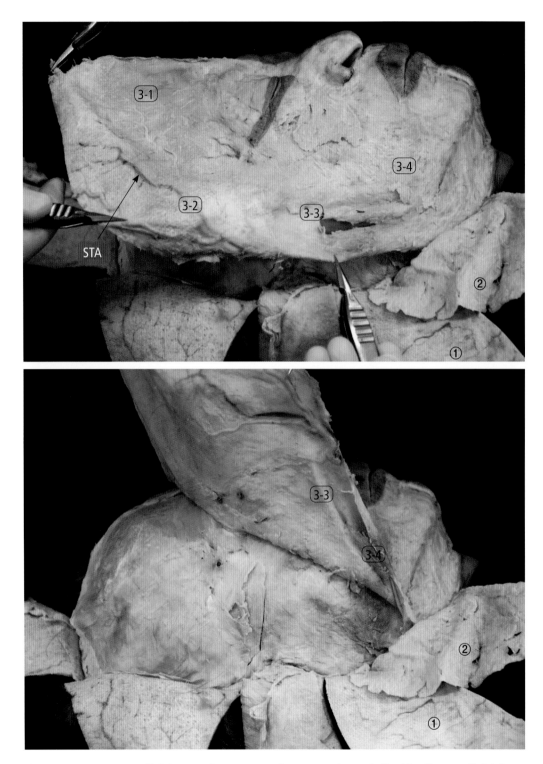

Fig. 2-3 Layer 3; Superficial Musculo-Aponeurotic System (SMAS) ① Skin ② Superficial fatty layer ③-1 Galeafrontalis ③-2 STF ③-3 SMAS ③-4 platysma

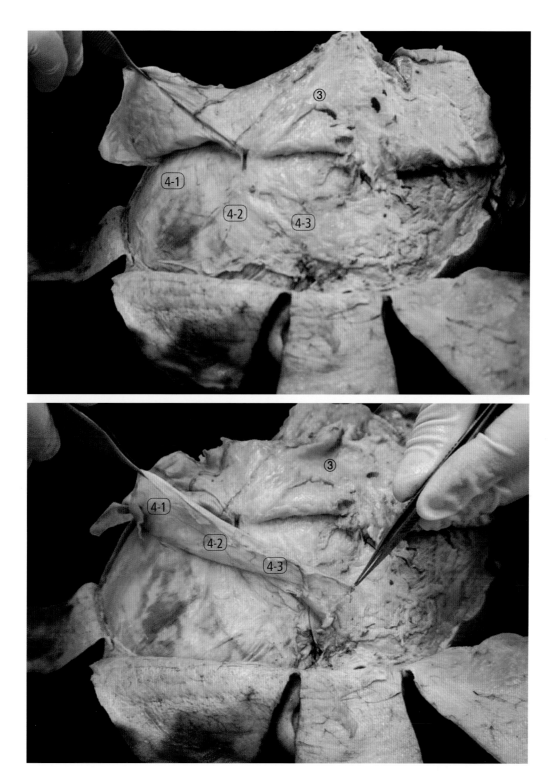

Fig. 2-4 **Layer 4; Loose areolar tissue** ③ SMAS ④-① **Subgaleal fascia** ④-② **Innominate fascia** ④-③ **Parotid temporal fascia**

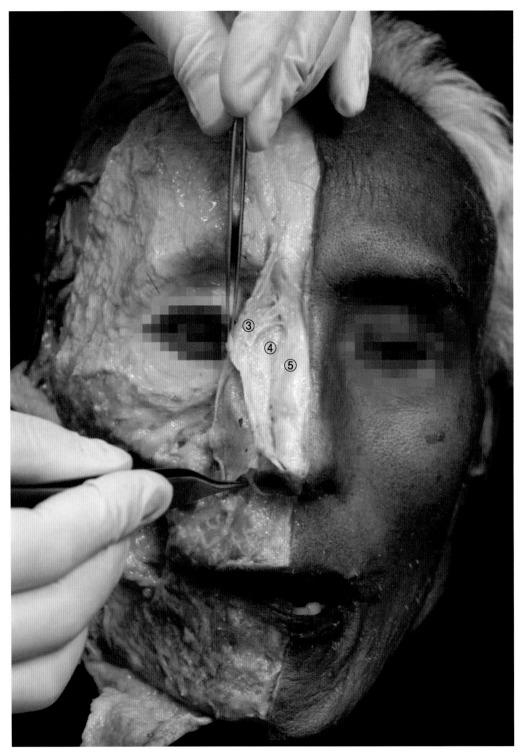

Fig. 2-5 **Layers of the Nose** ③ **Fibromuscular layer (SMAS)** ④ **Deep fatty layer** ⑤ **Periosteum and perichondrium**

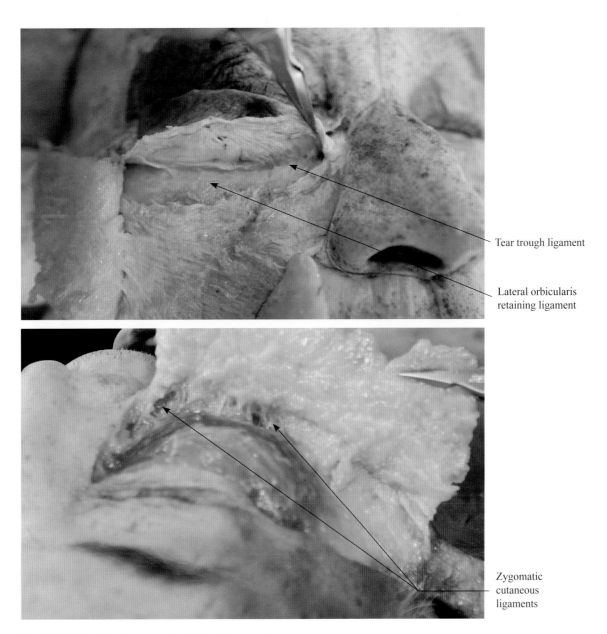

Tear trough ligament

Lateral orbicularis
retaining ligament

Zygomatic
cutaneous
ligaments

Fig. 2-6 Infraorbital groove; Retaining ligaments

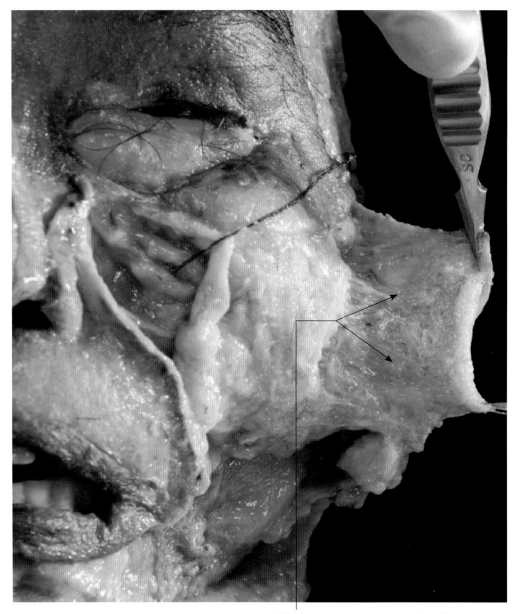

Masseteric cutaneous retaining ligaments

Fig. 2-7 Masseteric cutaneous retaining ligaments

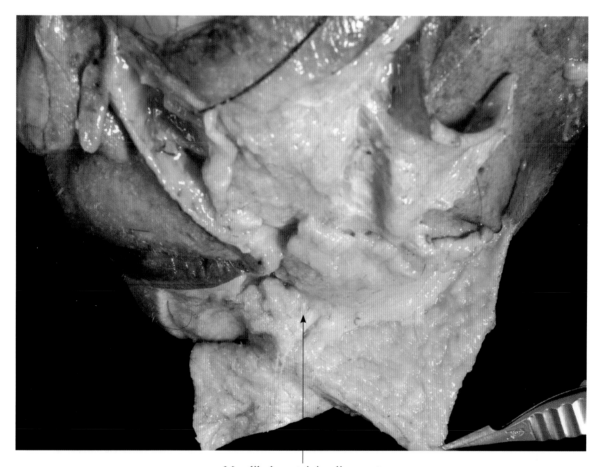

Mandibular retaining ligament

Fig. 2-8 Mandibular retaining ligament

Lateral orbital fat compartment   Inferior orbital fat compartment

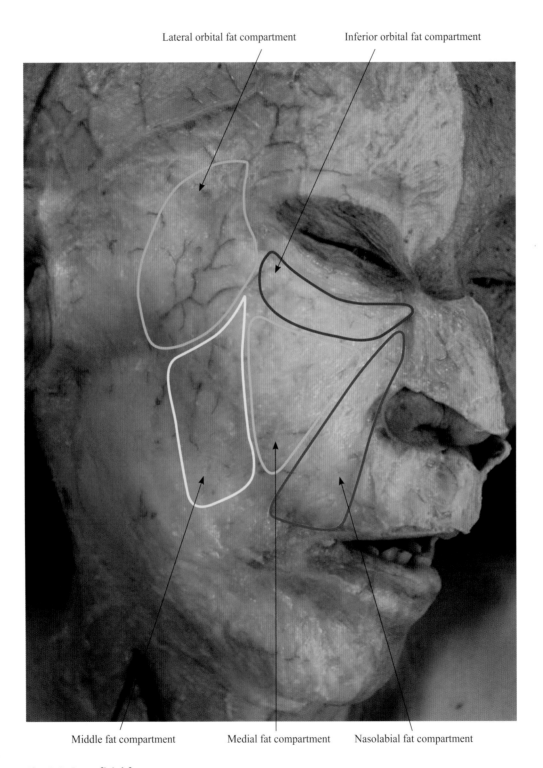

Middle fat compartment   Medial fat compartment   Nasolabial fat compartment

Fig. 2-9 **Superficial fat compartments**

2. 2 Muscles of the face

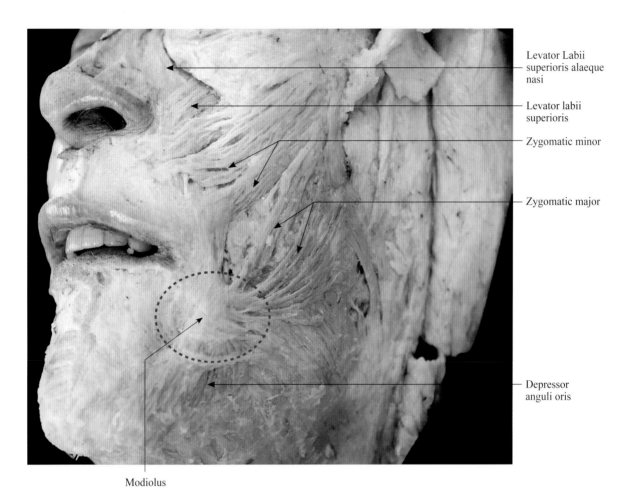

Levator Labii superioris alaeque nasi

Levator labii superioris

Zygomatic minor

Zygomatic major

Depressor anguli oris

Modiolus

Fig. 2-10 Facial muscles

2. 3 Facial vessels

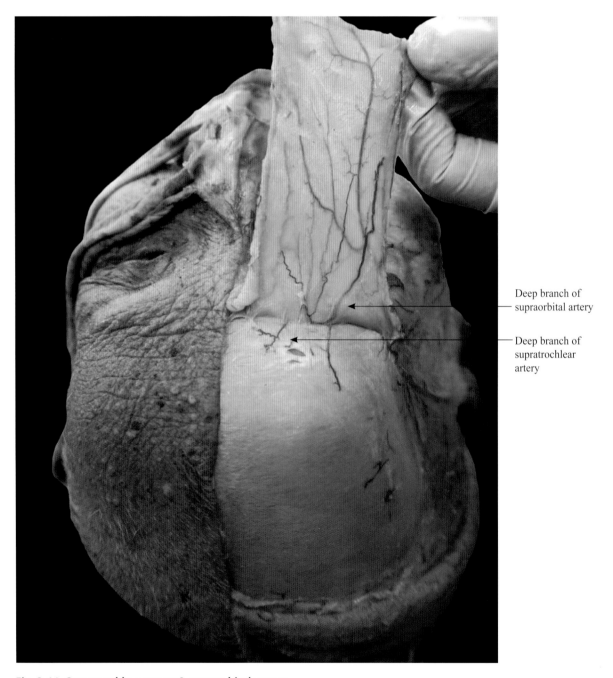

Deep branch of supraorbital artery

Deep branch of supratrochlear artery

Fig. 2-11 **Supratrochlear artery & supraorbital artery**

Sentinel (zygomaticotemporal) vein

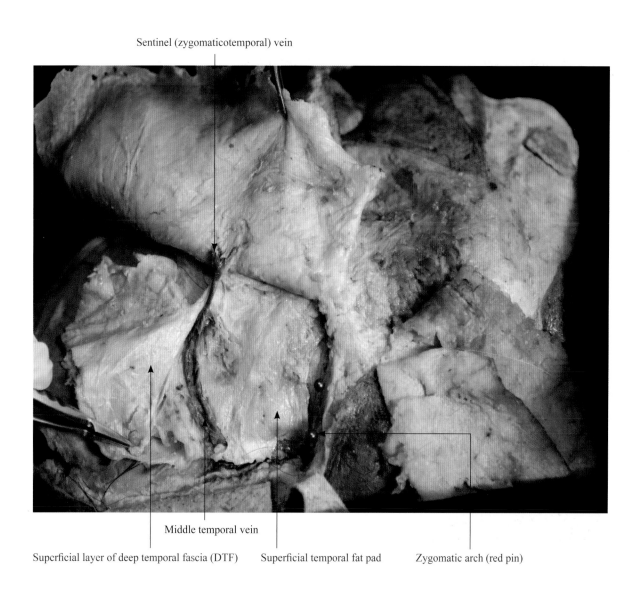

Superficial layer of deep temporal fascia (DTF)   Middle temporal vein   Superficial temporal fat pad   Zygomatic arch (red pin)

Fig. 2-12 Temple area vessels

Lateral nasal artery

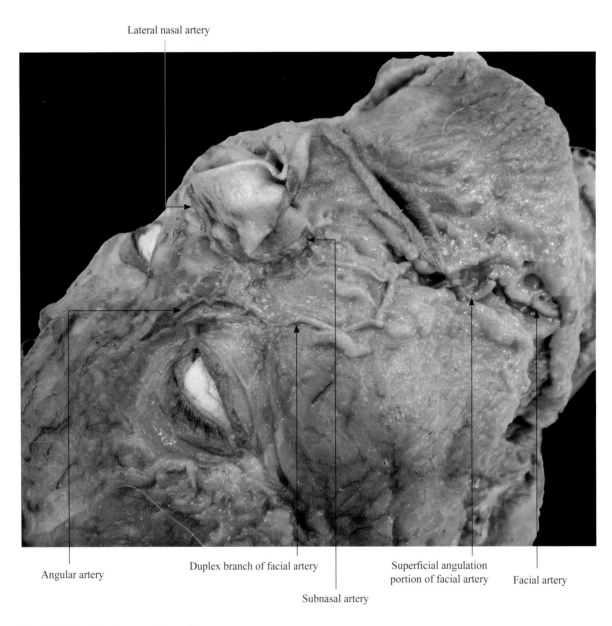

Angular artery

Duplex branch of facial artery

Subnasal artery

Superficial angulation
portion of facial artery

Facial artery

Fig. 2-13 Facial artery and branches

2. 4 Nerves of the face

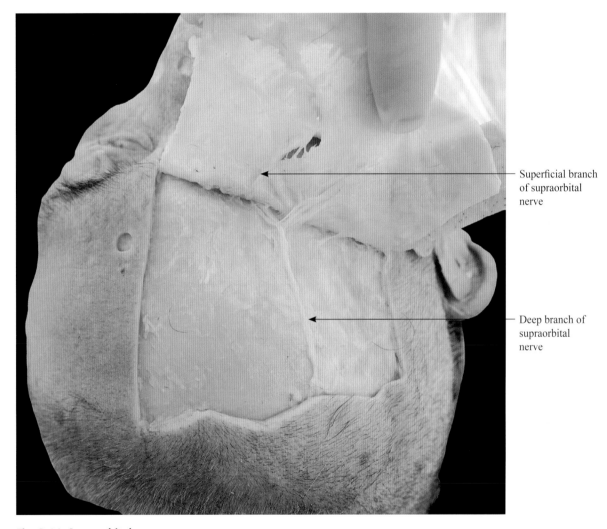

Superficial branch of supraorbital nerve

Deep branch of supraorbital nerve

Fig. 2-14 **Supraorbital nerve**

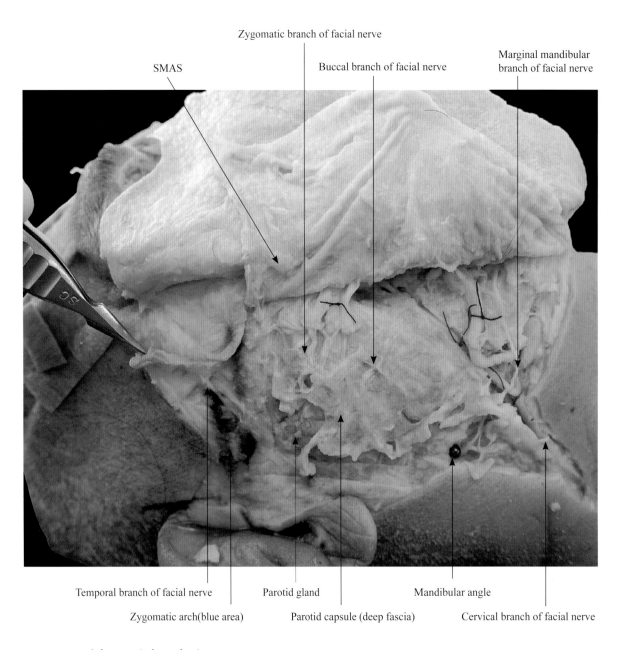

Zygomatic branch of facial nerve

SMAS

Buccal branch of facial nerve

Marginal mandibular
branch of facial nerve

Temporal branch of facial nerve

Zygomatic arch(blue area)

Parotid gland

Parotid capsule (deep fascia)

Mandibular angle

Cervical branch of facial nerve

Fig. 2-15 **Facial nerve (5 branches)**

Hyaluronic acid filler property

CHAPTER

03 Hyaluronic acid filler property

Won Lee, M.D., Ph.D., Plastic Surgeon

In this book, we described hyaluronic acid filler as hard filler or soft filler previously. In this chapter, we will discuss about hyaluronic acid filler property to understand injection of the proper filler at the appropriate site.

3. 1 Hyaluronic acid

Hyaluronic acid is a disaccharide in the skin, synovial fluid, and vitreous humors. Molecular structures are shown in Fig. 3-1.

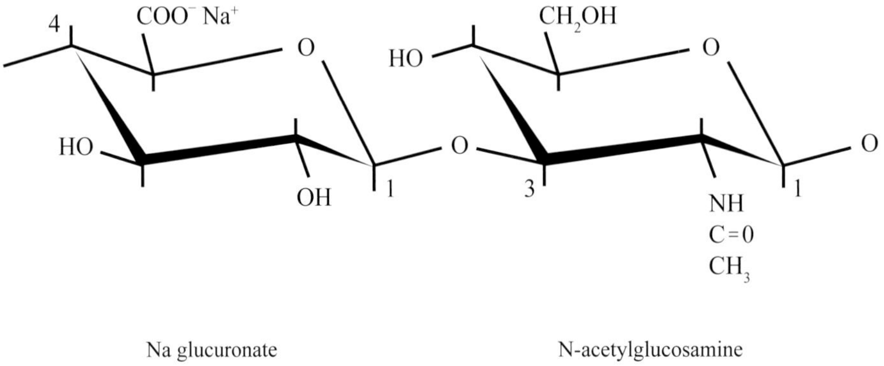
4
COO⁻ Na⁺
O
HO
CH2OH
O
HO
O
O
OH
1
3
NH
C=0
CH3
1
Na glucuronate
N-acetylglucosamine

Fig. 3-1 **Hyaluronic acid molecular structure**

3. 2 Hyaluronic acid manufacturing process

Hyaluronic acid filler is made by the following manufacturing process:

weight → dissolve → reaction → cutting → washing → sieving → filling → autoclaving

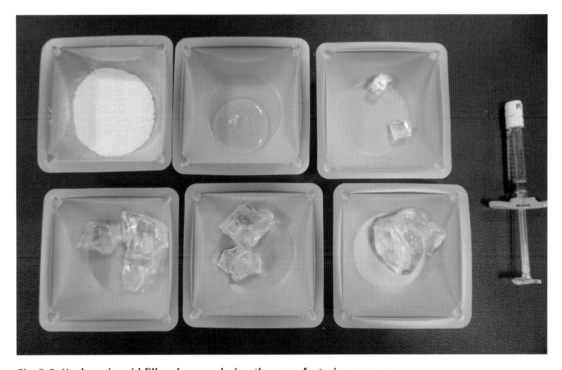

Fig. 3-2 **Hyaluronic acid filler changes during the manufacturing process**

3. 3 Property of hyaluronic acid filler

3. 3. 1 Biphasic versus monophasic

Generally, hyaluronic acid filler is divided into two categories. However, this classification is from manufacturing process differences and not scientific words. The most popular biphasic filler is known as Restylane®, and the most popular monophasic filler is known as Juvederm®.

3. 3. 2 Hyaluronic acid concentration

This means how much hyaluronic acid is in 1mL of filler. Many products contain 20 mg/mL.

Usually, 5.5 mg of hyaluronic acid is known to be equivalent to 1mL of water, so after injection of hyaluronic acid filler, swelling might develop because of attraction of adjacent water.

3. 3. 3 Particle size

Hyaluronic acid filler particle sizes are determined by the manufacturing process. Some products are divided into hard or soft filler by particle sizes.

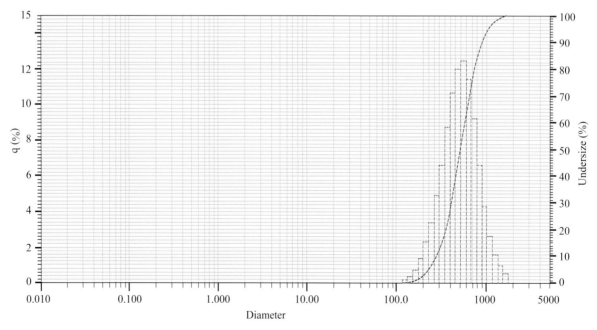

Fig. 3-3 Particle size: Chaeum®

3. 3. 4 Injection force

It is the parameter of how much power is needed to inject this specific filler. It should be tested with a same-diameter needle.

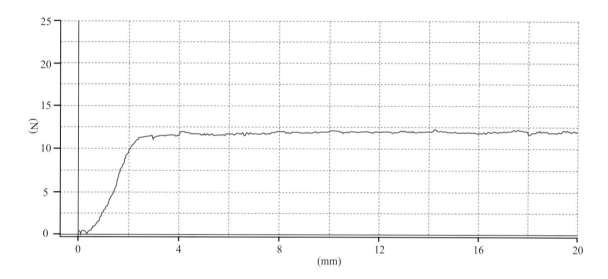

Fig. 3-4 Injection force (N) 27-G needle, hyaluronic acid filler

3. 3. 5 Rheology

Objective parameters of the filler are tested by a rheometer. This parameter shows us how hard or how sticky the filler is and more data.

Rheology parameters

G': elastic modulus, storage modulus

It is the parameter of deformation degree from external stress. When G' is high, the filler is relatively unlikely to deform. It has a slightly different meaning but indicates how hard it is.

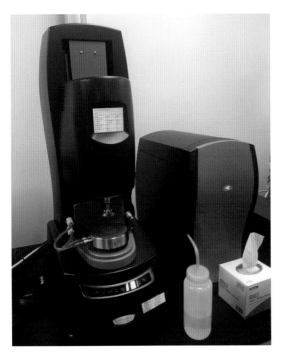

Fig. 3-5 Rheometer

Complex viscosity

It is the parameter of resistance. When the complex viscosity is high, the filler is relatively difficult to inject.

Cohesiveness

It is the objective parameter of how much the fillers aggregate each other. It is not a specific rheological term but is a very important parameter.

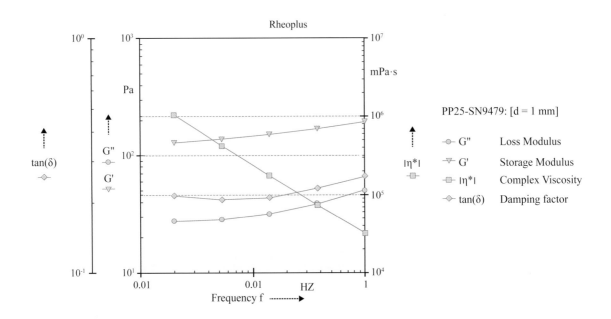

Fig. 3-6 Rheologic data of one hyaluronic acid filler. G′, G″, complex viscosity, tan δ

(Courtesy from Biomedical Dermatology 2018 Clinical application of a new hyaluronic acid filler based on its rheological properties of the anatomical site of injection. Won Lee et al. /doi.org/10.1186/s41702-018-0032-9)

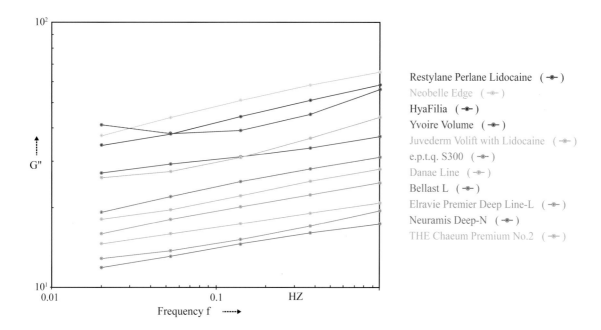

Fig. 3-7 Rheologic G′ data of various hyaluronic acid fillers. Hz: 0.02–1Hz at 25°C

(Courtesy from Dermatologic Surgery 2019 Practical guidelines for hyaluronic acid soft tissue filler applications in facial rejuvenation. Won Lee et al.)

Suggestive Readings

1. Lee W, Yoon J-H, Koh I-S, Oh W, Kim K-W, Yang E-J. Clinical application of a new hyaluronic acid filler based on its rheological properties and the anatomical site of injection. Biomedical Dermatology. 2018;2(1).

2. Yang B, Guo X, Zang H, Liu J. Determination of modification degree in BDDE-modified hyaluronic acid hydrogel by SEC/MS. Carbohydrate polymers. 2015;131:233-9.

3. Choi SC, Yoo MA, Lee SY, Lee HJ, Son DH, Jung J, et al. Modulation of biomechanical properties of hyaluronic acid hydrogels by crosslinking agents. Journal of biomedical materials research Part A. 2015;103(9):3072-80.

4. De Boulle K, Glogau R, Kono T, Nathan M, Tezel A, Roca-Martinez JX, et al. A review of the metabolism of 1,4-butanediol diglycidyl ether-crosslinked hyaluronic acid dermal fillers. Dermatologic surgery : official publication for American Society for Dermatologic Surgery [et al]. 2013;39(12):1758-66.

5. Tezel A, Fredrickson GH. The science of hyaluronic acid dermal fillers. Journal of cosmetic and laser therapy : official publication of the European Society for Laser Dermatology. 2008;10(1):35-42.

Equivalence Table: The Chaeum (Dermalax®) Series

	Lidocaine	Brand	Volume					
			0	1	2	3	4	5
Domestic (Korea) Chaeum	Without Lidocaine	Shape						Shape10
		Pure		No.1	No.2	No.3	No.4	
	With Lidocaine	Premium	Moist	No.1	No.2	No.3	No.4	
		Style		No.1	No.2	No.3	No.4	
Export	Without Lidocaine	Volus						Volus10
		Hyalsense		Fine	Ultra	Sub-Q		
		Demalax		Demalx	Deep	Implant		
		Revolax		Fine	Deep	Sub-Q		
		Dermaren		Fine	Deep	Sub-Q		
		JBPNanolink		Fine	Deep	Sub-Q		
	With Lidocaine	Hyalsense		Fine Plus	Ultra Plus	Sub-Q Plus		
		Demalax		Plus	Deep Plus	Implant Plus		
		Revigance		Plus	Deep Plus	Implant Plus		
		Revolax		Finew/L	Deepw/L	Sub-Qw/L		
		Dermaren		Finew/L	Deepw/L	Sub-Qw/L		
		JBPNanolink		Finew/L	Deepw/L	Sub-Qw/L		

CHAPTER **04**

Forehead

Gi-Woong Hong, M.D., Ph.D., Plastic Surgeon

4. 1. 1 Considerations before injection.

The boundary of the forehead is known to be from the trichion of the hairline to the eyebrow vertically and bilateral superior temporal septum (STS) of the temporal crest horizontally. Compared to Western people who have longer frontooccipital length and narrow skull, Oriental people have wider and shorter frontooccipital length skull. However, although they have larger horizontal width, the real forehead horizontal length is usually short. Moreover, since Oriental people tend to have smaller horizontal eye width, intercanthal distance tends to look greater than that in Western people. The forehead should be convex in shape and regular at the lateral view and have an S line upper face shape to show a soft facial image. Moreover, irregular forehead shape at the front view could make the forehead look shorter and create a stuffy image that needs improvement. A forehead with adequate convexity could make the face look smaller. Since Oriental people like small faces, augmentation of the forehead and correction of the glabella are adequate procedures for them. One concern is not to augment higher than the supraorbital ridge because the eyebrow and orbital area tend to be sunken and the nose also tends to be depressed.

Usually, the lower 2/3 of the forehead is depressed, and the region between the frontal eminence and supraorbital ridge is like to be depressed, which is usually classified into three types: central type, which is a depressed upper glabella; bilateral type, which is a depressed region above the eyebrow; and mixed type. The upper 1/3 is not likely to be sunken but is likely to have an abrupt angle, and there might be a total type, which is depressed lower and upper part.

Glabella depression has multiple causes. Skeletal depression would result in glabella depression. Soft tissue depression would also lead to glabella depression but is usually accompanied by a vertical wrinkle by glabellar frowning and a horizontal wrinkle by procerus muscle contraction. Wrinkles usually appear bilaterally but could also appear as a unilateral prominent vertical wrinkle (Fig. 4-1).

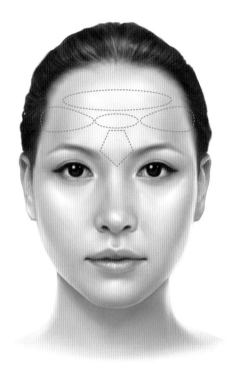

Forehead depression
lower 2/3 part of forehead : main depression
upper 1/3 part of forehead : minor depression
1) bilateral type
2) central type
3) mixed type
4) total type

Glabella depression
1) bone type
2) fat type
3) crease type
4) mixed type

Fig. 4-1 Types of forehead and glabella depression

Shallow wrinkles by dermal atrophy or minimal depression can be corrected by botulinum toxin and/or filler injections. However, deep wrinkles by long-term muscle contraction, subcutaneous fat depression, and scar-like wrinkles could not be corrected adequately, so it is important to predict the results. Furthermore, glabella depression tends to be accompanied by forehead depression, so it is better to provide an explanation to the patients and inject both areas simultaneously.

4. 1. 2 Anatomical considerations

Central and bilateral middle forehead compartments are located at the subcutaneous layer. Middle forehead compartments are connected to the lateral temporal cheek fat compartment laterally at the temple area, and STS is located between them. In injection at this layer, there are several problems such as superficial running arteries and big diameter veins; injection of hard consistency filler would result in irregularity and difficult molding because of the septum between compartments (Fig. 4-2).

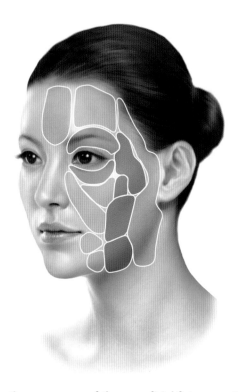

Facial fat pads rersorb over time
Resorption sequences (1~5)

1 (Red)	=	Superior and inferior orbital fat pad
2 (Green)	=	Medial cheek fat compartments
3 (Blue)	=	Lateral orbital fat and lateral cheek fat compartments
4 (Yellow)	=	Nasolabial and jowl fat compartments
5 (Pink)	=	Central and midline forehead compartments Lateral temporal-cheek fat compartments

Fig. 4-2 Resorption sequences of the superficial fat compartments

The frontalis muscle attaches to the eyebrow to pull it upward, and the antagonistic muscles are the procerus, corrugator and depressor supercilii, and orbicularis muscles, which pull the eyebrow downward. The frontalis muscle extends to the galea aponeurotica and is connected to the occipital muscle posteriorly. Laterally, it elongates to the STF crossing over the STS. There is a space between the frontalis muscle and bone, and deep fat compartments are seen at the lateral part of this space, but the medial part is

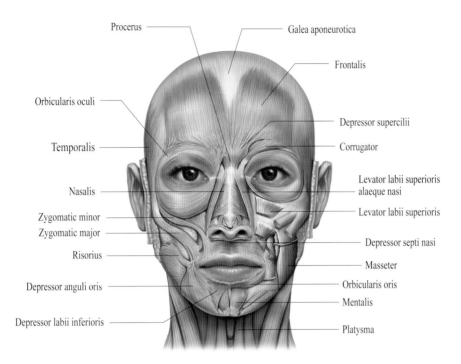

Procerus — Galea aponeurotica

Frontalis

Orbicularis oculi —

Depressor supercilii

Temporalis — Corrugator

Levator labii superioris
alaeque nasi

Nasalis — Levator labii superioris

Zygomatic minor —
Zygomatic major — Depressor septi nasi

Risorius — Masseter

Depressor anguli oris — Orbicularis oris

Mentalis

Depressor labii inferioris — Platysma

Fig. 4-3 **Muscles of the face**

almost not detected (Fig. 4-3).

The frontalis muscle bifurcates 3.5 cm above the superior orbital rim but divides into a higher level and sometimes does not bifurcate. Thus, there is a recommendation to inject botulinum toxin to the upper medial portion.

The corrugator supercilii muscle is located in the deepest part, which pulls the eyebrow downward and forms vertical glabella wrinkle and divides the transverse and oblique head but is not clinically important. It originates 1cm above the nasion and 3 mm lateral from midline and runs in a fan-shaped upward direction and attaches to the eyebrow skin. When we show a glabella frown, just lateral from wrinkle line is where the corrugator muscle attaches to the skin, and thickest part is approximately 2~3 mm in thickness and located between the medial canthus and midpupillary line.

The procerus originates between the nasal SMAS near the nasion and medial canthal region and runs upward and attaches to the skin between the eyebrows, and when it is contracted, it forms a horizontal wrinkle at the dorsum of the nose.

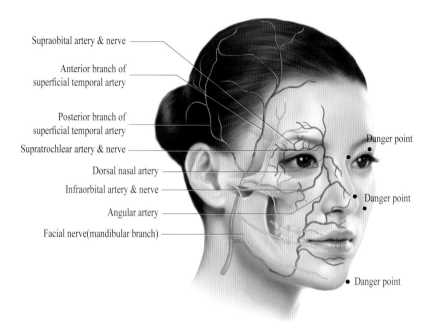

Fig. 4-4 **Blood supply of the lateral forehead area**

The superficial temporal artery divides into the frontal (anterior) and temporal (posterior) branches at the horizontal level of the superior orbital rim, and frontal branch runs in a superior medial 60° direction and meets the frontalis muscle lateral border at 1.5~2 cm above the eyebrow tail upper margin. It is located deeper to the STF at the level of the frontalis muscle lateral margin and runs superficially in the subcutaneous layer at the level of the vertical line of the lateral canthus, so it is important not to tear the vessel when injecting superficially. The facial nerve frontal branch also runs across the temple area to the frontalis muscle 1~1.5 cm above the lateral eyebrow end (Fig. 4-4).

The supratrochlear artery and nerve perforates supratrochlear notch or foramen of the medial orbit at the level of vertical line of the medial canthus. The supratrochlear artery divides into the superficial and deep branches. The deep branch runs deeply along the periosteum, and the superficial branch perforates the frontalis muscle 1.5 cm above the superior orbital rim and runs in the subcutaneous layer. The superficial branch is the main branch of the supratrochlear artery.

This superficial branch of the supratrochlear artery is located along the glabellar frown line (corrugator crease), and the central forehead artery can be located along the central forehead crease, so care should be taken when correcting these wrinkles.

The supraorbital artery and nerve perforate supraorbital foramen, which is located at vertical line of the medial limbus, and run between the transverse and oblique heads of the corrugator muscle and perforate the frontalis muscle at the superficial branch (Fig. 4-5).

Frontalis muscle perforation pathways of the supratrochlear artery and nerve and supraorbital artery and nerve are variable, so care should be taken, and since the supratrochlear artery runs superficially than the supraorbital artery, subcutaneous injection in the glabellar area should be cautiously performed to prevent subdermal plexus damage and skin necrosis (Fig. 4-6).

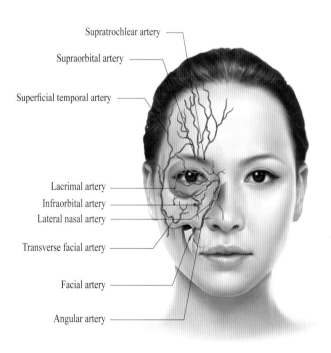

Supratrochlear artery

Supraorbital artery

Superficial temporal artery

Lacrimal artery
Infraorbital artery
Lateral nasal artery

Transverse facial artery

Facial artery

Angular artery

Fig. 4-5 Blood supply of forehead and glabella

Usually, forehead depression is noticed above the supraorbital ridge, and arteries are already likely to perforate the muscles and run superficially in this location, so it is relatively safe to inject at the supra-periosteal layer.

Ocular swelling might develop because the filler could migrate through the weakened orbital retaining ligament (ORL) after injection, which is located 2~3 mm above the superior orbital rim and works as barrier between the forehead and orbit. Another reason could be because the excessive ROOF pad could be a space for migration. Therefore, it is not recommended to inject near the supraorbital ridge and a small amount of soft filler to the subdermal layer.

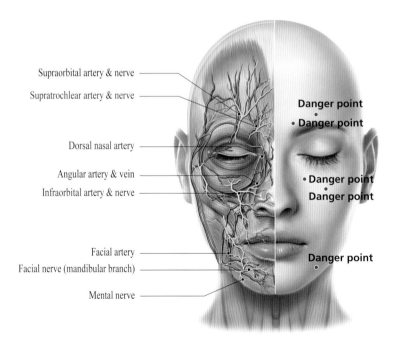

Supraorbital artery & nerve

Supratrochlear artery & nerve

Danger point
Danger point

Dorsal nasal artery

Angular artery & vein

Danger point

Infraorbital artery & nerve

Danger point

Facial artery

Facial nerve (mandibular branch)

Danger point

Mental nerve

Fig. 4-6 Danger points: high-risk areas

4. 1. 3 Injection technique

4. 1. 3. 1 Forehead

The entry point is the upper margin of the lateral part of the eyebrow where borderline of forehead and temple at the bilateral type or not much central depressed mixed type of forehead depression. After puncturing with the needle, insert the cannula, perforating the frontalis muscle, and place the cannula under the muscle. Check the periosteum, and move the cannula tip gently. The cannula tip can be moved easily because of the submuscular space. Since the forehead is not of a completely flat shape, the cannula tip should proceed in a fan-type technique, feeling the periosteum. When approaching the desired location, filler injection should be performed in a retrograde fanning technique at the submuscular plane (Fig. 4-7).

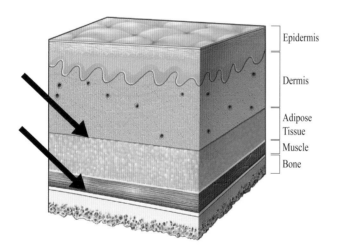

Epidermis

Dermis

Adipose Tissue

Muscle

Bone

▷ Submuscular injection for volume
Perlane or subQ: 1~2 mL
SubQ: 23 G cannula
Perlane: 27 G cannula

▷ Subdermal injection to improve the
depressed wrinkle line and to compensate
the deficient area to make even surface
- Restylane lidocaine 0.5~1 mL
: 30 G nano needle

Fig. 4-7 Forehead: Injection plane, Products, Injection volume and accessories

Additional entry point could be made at central-type depression where the midline puncture point between glabella and central depressed forehead area is located. The entry point should be slightly lateral to the midline to avoid the central forehead artery. Perforate the frontalis muscle and locate the cannula tip at the submuscular plane. Then, inject the filler using retrograde fanning, cross-hatching, and droplet techniques.

Upper forehead depression is seen at total-type depression. The entry point should be made at the hairline vertical from the midpupillary line. Moreover, injection should be performed at the submuscular plane (Fig. 4-8).

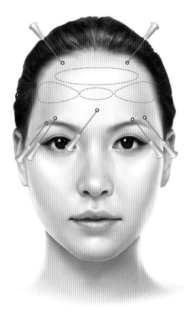

Injection entry points forehead
- Lower 2/3 part (main depression)
  1) upper margin of lateral eyebrow
  2) upper margin of eyebrow between lateral limbus and lateral canthus around border of forehead and temple
  3) inferior mid-point of central depression upper 1/3 part : anterior hairline point

Injection technique
- Retrograde horizontal fanning and crossing
- Droplet technique to smooth out the surface

Fig. 4-8 Forehead: Injection points and techniques for cannula

After volume augmentation, it is recommended to inject the soft filler at the subdermal layer to cover irregularity or borderline of the area not injected (Fig. 4-9, 4-10).

It is recommended to inject botulinum toxin together and frontalis muscle action could result in dynamic wrinkles because injected filler would migrate or affect longevity of the filler. When there are static wrinkles that are not affected by the frontalis muscle, it is recommended to inject the soft filler in the dermal layer by fern-leaf or duck-walk technique.

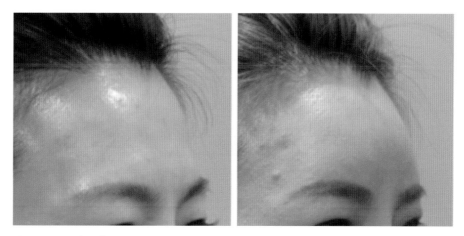

Fig. 4-9 **Forehead augmentation: pre-and post-injection**

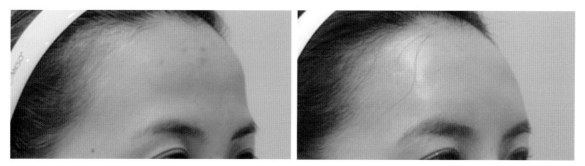

Fig. 4-10 **Forehead augmentation: pre-and post-injection**

4. 1. 3. 2 Glabella

In injecting in glabella area depression, it is recommended to make an entry point at the point between the forehead depression and glabella area but slightly lateral to the midline as described before. Perforate the glabella area muscles, and inject at the submuscular layer using retrograde fanning, droplet, and linear threading techniques. After volumizing, inject the soft filler at the dermal or subdermal layer to make a smooth contour (Fig. 4-11).

Glabellar depression is usually formed at the glabellar frown line, which is contraction of the corrugator supercilii muscle, so it is recommended to inject botulinum toxin and filler at each wrinkle line (Fig. 4-12).

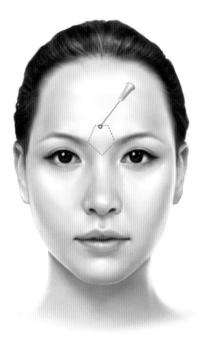

Injection entry point for glabella
• slightly lateral to superior mid-point of area requiring volume

Injection technique
• Retrograde fanning
• Droplet and linear threading to smooth out the surface

Fig. 4-11 Glabella: injection point and techniques

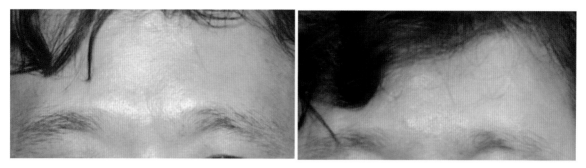

Fig. 4-12 **Glabella depression correction: pre-and post-injection**

Usually, the supratrochlear artery superficial branch tends to run inside or above the muscle; therefore, injecting at the subcutaneous layer is dangerous. It is recommended to inject a soft filler at the dermal or subdermal layer (Fig. 4-13).

When injecting at the dermal or subdermal layer, it is recommended to inject the filler not using the linear threading technique but the fern-leaf technique, which is injecting the filler at the lateral side perpendicular to the wrinkle, or duck-walk technique, which is injecting 60° lateral to the wrinkle. Moreover, the filler can be injected at the lateral side of the wrinkle, so it is better to use the pinching and/or holding technique and stretching technique to inject at the exact location of the wrinkle. These methods are effective in making a flat contour. Since arteries tend to run along the wrinkles, vascular compromise could occur when injection is performed parallel to the wrinkle.

In glabellar frowning, the procerus muscle also contracts and forms horizontal wrinkles at the dorsum of the nose. It is recommended to inject botulinum toxin, and a filler can be used together. However, since there is an intercanthal vein in 70% of Oriental people in this area, it is also recommended to inject the filler perpendicular to the wrinkle or in a 60° direction. It is better to use a soft filler and inject at the dermal or subdermal layer and, if volume needed, inject at the submuscular layer.

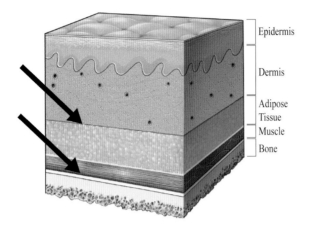

Epidermis

Dermis

Adipose
Tissue

Muscle

Bone

• Submuscular injection for volume
Perlane or SubQ: 0.5~1 mL
Perlane: 27 G cannula
SubQ: 23 G cannula

• Subdermal injection to improve the depressed wrinkle
line and to compensate the deficient area to make even
surface
- Restylane lidocaine 0.3~0.5 mL
  : 30 G nano needle
- Be cautious when injecting into glabellar frown line
due to supratrochlear artery branch
- Beware of central forehead artery on the midline forehead crease

Fig. 4-13 Glabella: Injection plane, Products, Injection volume and accessories

Suggestive Readings

1. Costin BR, Plesec TP, Sakolsatayadorn N, Rubinstein TJ, McBride JM, Perry JD. Anatomy and histology of the frontalis muscle. Ophthalmic plastic and reconstructive surgery. 2015;31(1):66-72.
2. Jones D. Volumizing the face with soft tissue fillers. Clinics in plastic surgery. 2011;38(3):379-90, v.
3. Pessa JE, Rohrich RJ. Facial Topography: Clinical Anatomy of the Face: Quality Medical Pub.; 2012.
4. Rohrich RJ, Pessa JE. The fat compartments of the face: anatomy and clinical implications for cosmetic surgery. Plastic and reconstructive surgery. 2007;119(7):2219-27; discussion 28-31.
5. Wu W, Carlisle I, Huang P, Ribe N, Russo R, Schaar C, et al. Novel administration technique for large-particle stabilized hyaluronic acid-based gel of nonanimal origin in facial tissue augmentation. Aesthetic plastic surgery. 2010;34(1):88-95.

Hyung-Ik Baik, M.D., Plastic Surgeon

Forehead 4-2

CHAPTER

4. 2. 1 Design

The preinjection design is very important because the forehead is relatively wide and irregular in shape. Local anesthesia injection could result in an irregular shape, and the filler injection site could be uneven. The preinjection design varies depending on the patient's demand. When injecting the whole forehead, the design would be as follows. Horizontal borderline of the forehead would be the border between the forehead and temple. Depending on supraorbital ridge protrusion, the lower border would be near the eyebrows or above the protruded area. The upper border would depend on the hairline, and injection could be performed into or below the hairline. The protruded and depressed areas should be marked before injection, and the filler amount should be virtually distributed.

4. 2. 2 Anesthesia

Regional anesthesia blocking the supratrochlear nerve and supraorbital nerve would be performed. However, forehead augmentation should be done with caution because of long procedure time and possibility of surface irregularity. The author like to perform local anesthesia infiltration because of reduction in patient's discomfort of feeling the cannula or the needle end contacting the skull. Five entry points are injected with local anesthesia, and using a 23G 50 mm cannula, the whole area of the forehead is infiltrated by 1% lidocaine mixed with 1:200,000 epinephrine. Less than 3mL lidocaine is used.

4. 2. 3 Technique
4. 2. 3. 1 Cannula

Using a 23G 50 mm cannula, five entry points are used, and the injected areas are overlapped using the fanning technique. First, locate the cannula tip, and inject the filler by pulling the cannula backward.

61

Enough time is needed because not too much filler is injected in one region. The supraperiosteal or sub-galeal layer is used.

4. 2. 3. 2 Total volume should not exceed 3 mL

4. 2. 3. 3 Progression: pre-and post-injection photograph

Infiltrated local anesthesia would be absorb within a few hours or at least 1 day after filler injection, but swelling could develop due to local anesthesia and filler injection. It is recommended to observe progression after 1 week. However, the patient should be encouraged to visit the clinic when any doubtful changes are observed after injection.

4. 2. 3. 4 Cautions

Extreme caution should be taken at the level of supratrochlear/supraorbital notch or foramen because the supratrochlear/supraorbital arteries did not perforate the frontalis muscle yet and are deeply located at the supraperiosteal layer, which is the same layer of filler injection.

4. 2. 3. 5 Complications and management

Swelling near the eye, glabella, and nose might develop 1 day after injection, and this might be caused by local anesthesia infiltration at the lower portion due to filler injection near the eyebrow. Cold pack is helpful.

Scalp paresthesia or neuralgia would develop when the supraorbital or supratrochlear nerve is damaged during the procedure, and symptomatic treatment is recommended until recovery.

Within 2~3 days after injection, when there is redness and tenderness, skin necrosis should be considered and managed immediately. Hyaluronidase should be injected considering the supratrochlear and supraorbital artery location. Vasodilation procedures such as gentle massage are helpful.

Forehead augmentation at a glance

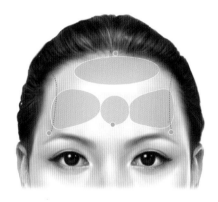 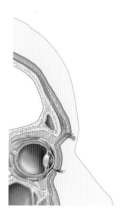

• **Dr. Gi-Woong Hong (Plastic Surgeon)'s technique: forehead**

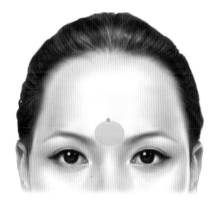 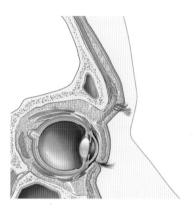

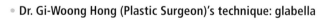

• **Dr. Gi-Woong Hong (Plastic Surgeon)'s technique: glabella**

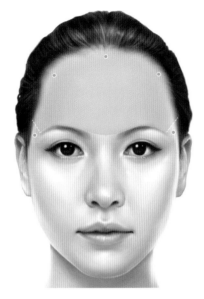

• **Dr. Hyung-Ik Baik (Plastic Surgeon)'s technique: forehead**

	Dr. Hong: forehead (PS)	Dr. Hong: glabella (PS)	Dr. Baik (PS)
Needle/cannula	23G cannula Hard filler for augmentation soft filler for smooth surface	23G cannula: depressed area 30G needle: wrinkle	23G cannula
Unilateral amount	Hard filler: 1.5~2 mL Soft filler: 0.5~1 mL	Depression: hard filler 0.5~1 mL Wrinkle: most soft filler 　　　　　0.3~0.5 mL	3 mL
Elasticity The Chaeum	Hard filler: No.3 Soft filler: No.2	Hard filler: No.3 Soft filler: No.1	No.3
Anesthesia	EMLA cream Local lidocaine at the entry point	EMLA cream Local lidocaine at the entry point	Local lidocaine Regional anesthesia
Techniques	Retrograde horizontal fanning and crossing technique: 　wide augmentation Droplet technique: 　partial augmentation	Retrograde horizontal fanning and crossing technique Droplet technique Fern-leaf or duck-walk tech- nique: wrinkle	Fan technique
Layer	Hard filler: submuscularlayer Soft filler: subdermal layer	Hard filler: submuscular layer Soft filler: dermal or superficial 　　　　　subdermal layer	Supraperiosteal layer

Temple

5-1 Temple

Hyung-Ik Baik, M.D., Plastic Surgeon

5. 1. 1 Design

In deciding the depressed area, draw a virtual line between the zygomatic arch and skull. Draw an upper and lower borderline and from lateral part of the orbital rim to the hairline.

5. 1. 2 Anesthesia

Local anesthesia of 1% lidocaine mixed with 1:200,000 epinephrine is injected at the entry point. Inject the whole temple area using a 23G cannula.

5. 1. 3 Technique

5. 1. 3. 1 Cannula

Using a 23G 50 mm cannula, approach the layer between the STF and DTF, and inject the filler using the fanning technique. Always locate the cannula tip at the desired area first, and inject the filler using the retrograde injection technique. The entry point should be considered by superficial temporal artery location. However, the entry point location is not so important because the main vessel is not located at the punctured site. It is more important to not vascularly compromised the cannula location or filler injection layer from a vascular perspective. An easily and evenly injected entry point would be slightly lower than the temple lower border vertically and at the center of the temple horizontally. Even if the cannula tip is blunt, it is not difficult to perforate the STF and locate the cannula tip between STF and DTF. The advantages are as follows: First, important structures such as the superficial temporal artery and temporal branch of the facial nerve are protected by the STF, so it is relatively safe to inject in this layer rather than in the subcutaneous layer. Second, it easily makes the surface smooth than injecting in the subcutaneous layer. Compared with subtemporalis muscle injection, it has the same effect but less amount of filler is used. Another possible layer might be between the superficial and deep layers of the DTF, but it is difficult to distribute the filler evenly. Moreover, the middle zygomatic vein is located, so it is recommended not to inject in this layer except when injecting in a depressed area just above the zygomatic arch.

5. 1. 3. 2 Total amount would be approximately 1 mL on each side

5. 1. 3. 3 Progression: pre- and post-injection photograph

Swelling easily resolves, so it is recommended to follow up within 1 week if there are no severe problems.

5. 1. 3. 4 Cautions

Injection should be gentle and smooth because, if there is bleeding, the periocular area would have severe bruising.

5. 1. 3. 5 Complications and management

Bruising might develop, so supportive treatment should be performed.

5-2 Temple

Gi-Woong Hong, M.D., Ph.D., Plastic Surgeon

5. 2. 1 Considerations before injection

The temple is a concave area below the superior temporal line (STL) or STS where the temporalis muscle originates. Oriental people have prominent zygoma and zygomatic arch, so temple hollowness is likely to be more prominent because of volume loss during the aging process. Thus, facial impression would be improved when volumizing the temple area and making a smooth contour between the lateral skull line and zygomatic arch.

5. 2. 2 Anatomical considerations

Temple base consists of the temporal bone and is called the "temporal fossa." The temporalis muscle is located at this fossa, and above the muscle, there are two layers of fascia. The STF or temporoparietal fascia (TPF) covers the superficial temporal artery and vein and is connected to the galea aponeurotica at the forehead and SMAS at the midface. The deep fascia is called the DTF, temporalis fascia, or temporalis muscle fascia and starts at the STS, and as it runs downwards it divides into the superficial and deep layers, and two layers fuse together 1cm above the zygomatic arch or do not fuse and cover it. Multiple layers make several spaces. The buccal fat pad temporal extension, DTFP, is located between the temporalis muscle and DTF. Superficial temporal fat pad (STFP) is located between the superficial and deep layers of the DTF. It hangs 3~4 cm above the zygomatic arch. The upper and lower temporal compartment is divided by the inferior temporal septum (ITS) and located between the STF and DTF (Table 5-1).

The upper temporal compartment is surrounded by the STS and ITS, which are elongations of temporal and supraorbital ligamentous adhesions. It is composed of soft tissue without important vessel or nerve, so it is a safe region of anchoring site when thread lifting. The lower temporal compartment is

Table 5-1 Layers of temple compared to other layers

Basic layer	Midface	Temples
skin	skin	skin
subcutaneous tissue	superficical fat compartment	lateral temporal cheek fat
musculo aponeurotic layer	SMAS	superficial temporal fascia (STF) or temporoparietal fascia (TPF)
loose areolar tissue (LAT)	deep fat compartment	upper temporal compartment (UTC) or innominate fascia lower temporal compartment (LTC) or fibrofatty extension, parotid temporal fascia (PTF)
periosteum	facial muscles	superficial and deep layer of deep temporal fascia (DTF) or temporalis fascia (TF)

a triangular-shaped area below the ITS, and fat tissues are located at the lower part near the zygomatic arch region. This lower area is where important vessels and nerves are located, such as the facial nerve temporal branch, zygomaticotemporal nerve (ZTN) medial and lateral branch, and sentinel vein. The facial nerve temporal branch is likely to run parallel to the ITS border, but variation exists.

The temple area is supplied by the superficial and deep temporal arteries. The superficial temporal artery branches from the external carotid artery and supplies the temple and lateral forehead. The deep temporal artery branches from the maxillary artery (external carotid artery branch) and supplies the temple. The superficial temporal artery runs vertically along the preauricular crease just medial to the ear tragus, and at the level of horizontal line of the superior orbital rim, it divides into the anterior and posterior branches. The anterior branch runs in a 60° superomedial direction covered by the STF and meets the frontalis lateral margin 1.5~2 cm above the lateral eyebrow upper margin and runs superficially at the level of vertical line of the lateral canthus (Fig. 5-1).

The facial nerve temporal branch runs parallel to the ITS. Usually, it is located inferomedial than the STA anterior branch. Pitanguy's line is a virtual line of the facial nerve that is from 0.5 cm below the tragus to 1.5 cm above the eyebrow lateral margin. After perforating the parotid gland, the temporal branch perforates the parotid-masseteric fascia and crosses the zygomatic arch. Then, it runs superficially at the undersurface of the STF, so care should be taken when running the cannula superficially.

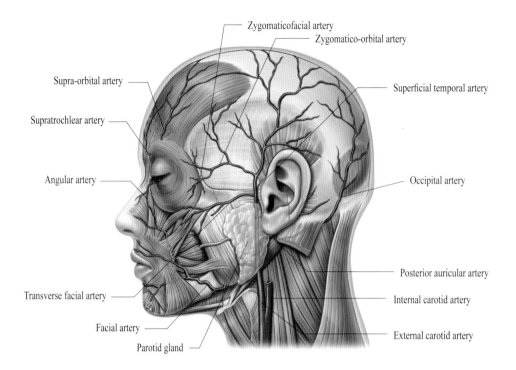

Fig. 5-1 Superficial temporal artery

Usually, the temporal branch runs superficially from 2~3 cm above the zygomatic arch to 1~1.5 cm lateral to the lateral orbital rim (Fig. 5-2).

The sentinel and middle temporal veins are one of the largest facial veins, and care should be taken because injection of the filler to the venous drainage might lead to cavernous sinus thrombosis or pulmonary embolism. The middle temporal vein is located at the STFP, which is located between the superficial and deep layers of the DTF. The middle temporal vein is 5~10 mm in diameter and located 2 cm above the upper border of zygomatic arch and drains to the superficial temporal vein. Filler injected into the internal jugular vein can result in pulmonary embolism, and a case of pulmonary fat embolism due to microfat injection was reported (Fig. 5-3).

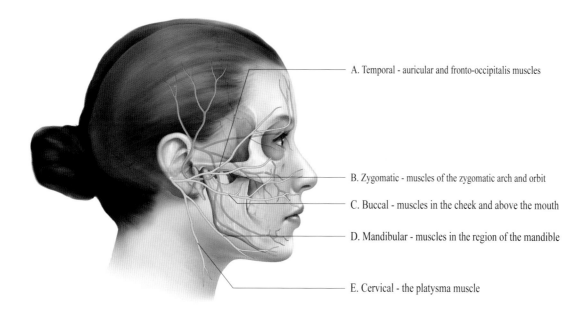

A. Temporal - auricular and fronto-occipitalis muscles

B. Zygomatic - muscles of the zygomatic arch and orbit

C. Buccal - muscles in the cheek and above the mouth

D. Mandibular - muscles in the region of the mandible

E. Cervical - the platysma muscle

Fig. 5-2 Facial motor nerves innervate the facial expression muscles

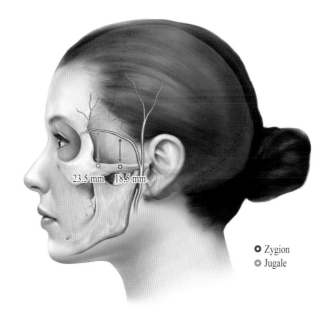

23.5 mm   18.5 mm

○ Zygion
○ Jugale

Fig. 5-3 Middle temporal vein

The sentinel vein, also called medial zygomaticotemporal vein, is a branch of the internal maxillary vein and 2~3 mm in diameter. Perpendicularly, it perforates the temporalis muscle and DTF and STF, and the location of perforation is 5mm lateral to the frontozygomatic suture line, which is 2.5 mm lateral to the lateral canthus. It can be seen as purple in color between the STF and DTF when performing face lift operation. After perforating the STF, it branches into the lateral eyebrow and temporal crest branches in the subcutaneous layer and can be seen when performing higher venous pressure procedures such as Valsalva maneuver. Sometimes, after temple augmentation by filler injection, this vessel might be seen more prominently. The sentinel vein is a kind of landmark structure, in which we would find the facial nerve temporal branch beneath it. Actually, the facial nerve temporal branch runs parallel to the ITS, and the sentinel vein runs below it, so some physicians insist that it could not be an indicator. Clinically, the sentinel vein usually communicates with the middle temporal vein, but some communicate with the periorbital vein and meet with the supratrochlear and supraorbital veins and might communicate with the cavernous sinus, so cavernous sinus thrombosis could develop during filler injection. In the region where the sentinel vein perforates the fascia, the facial nerve branch also runs superficially, and this region is called the caution zone. When we draw a line from the auricular helical root to superior orbit in-

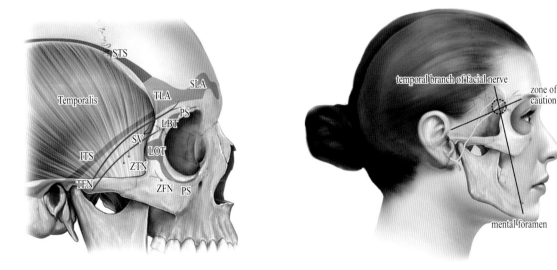

Fig. 5-4 Relationship of temporal branch of facial nerve(TFN) & sentinel vein

ner margin, the point with lateral orbital rim outer margin and 1 cm diameter circle is the caution zone, and it is where two structures are located (Fig. 5-4).

5. 2. 3 Technique

5. 2. 3. 1 Plane

Temporalis muscle volume and/or STFP volume can be decreased due to congenital conditions or weight loss, and also the DTFP volume can be decreased due to reduction in buccal fat pad during the aging process. There are multiple potential spaces of filler injection. The subcutaneous layer does not have enough fat tissues and might have irregular contour after injection. In cases with few depressions, it is recommended to inject between the STF and DTF compartment. When desiring to inject a large volume, it is recommended to inject at the STFP, between the superficial and deep layers of the DTF, or at the subtemporalis muscle layer. Injection at the DTFP is quite difficult, and injection into the temporalis muscle may damage the deep temporal artery and vein branches and also decrease longevity due to muscle action (Fig. 5-5).

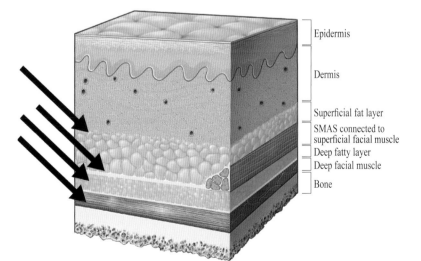

Epidermis

Dermis

Superficial fat layer
SMAS connected to superficial facial muscle
Deep fatty layer
Deep facial muscle
Bone

Injection plane
- Subfascial injection : between the STF (TPF) and DTF by cannula
- Superf. temporal fat pad (STFP) injection between superf. and deep layer of DTF by cannula
- submuscular area injection by needle when fat pad layer is scarce
- SubQ 1~2 mL for each area 23G needle or cannula if necessary, 0.5~1 mL restylane lidocaine subdermal injection to even the shoulder margin of the augmented area

Fig. 5-5 Temples: injection plane and products

73

5. 2. 3. 2 Point

Usually, the anterior 2/3 is likely to be depressed in the temple area. The recommended entry point would be the vertical line of the lateral canthus eyebrow with the uppermost point almost at the border of the forehead and temple. This entry point can avoid the superficial temporal artery anterior and facial nerve temporal branches. The venous branch should be avoided when it is seen under the skin. The first resistance after inserting the cannula at the entry point would be the STF, which is quite easy to puncture. The second resistance is the DTF, which is very hard, so the cannula could be approached between the two layers. Inject the filler at the upper and lower temporal compartments. Considering the ITS and approaching parallel to the ITS could avoid important vessels and nerves that are located under the ITS (Fig. 5-6).

When there is severe sunken temple, it is likely depressed above the zygomatic arch area. When injecting a large volume, it is recommended to inject between the superficial and deep layers of the DTF or at the subtemporalis muscle layer. Draw a 1.5 cm diameter virtual circle above the zygomatic arch upper margin and lateral orbital rim lateral margin, and injecting in this circle area would avoid the facial

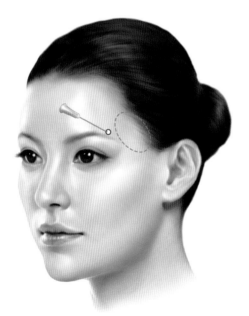

1st Injection entry point for anterior main depression
• upper margin of eyebrow on lateral canthal line around the border of forehead and temple

Injection technique
• Retrograde horizontal fanning technique

Fig. 5-6 Temples: Injection point and techniques for mild depression

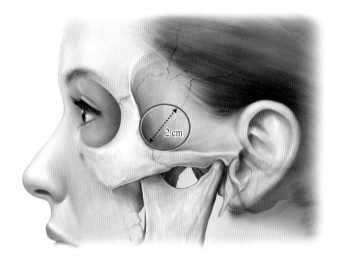

Fig. 5-7 Temples: Injection point and techniques for main depression

Circle with a 2 cm diameter along the border line of the upper margin of the zygomatic arch and the lateral margin of lateral orbital rim

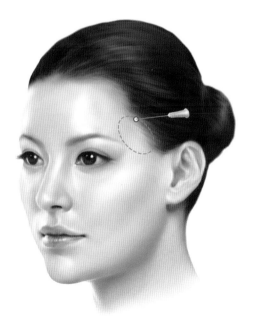

2nd Injection entry point for posterior depression, if necessary
• Anterior hairline point (about 1cm above eyebrow level)

Injection technique
• Retrograde horizontal fanning technique

Fig. 5-8 Temples: Injection point and techniques for posterior depression

nerve branch, ZTN, sentinel vein, and middle temporal vein (Fig. 5-7).

When injecting at the STFP, it is easy to perforate the STF first, then resistance at the DTF should be felt. In puncture, the next resistance is the perforating DTF superficial layer and hard resistance is the DTF deep layer. Gentle injection can be performed between the superficial and deep layers of the DTF where the STFP is located. The cannula tip should feel the DTF deep layer during injection and should not cross 2 cm above the zygomatic arch to avoid the middle zygomatic vein. The rest of the region is not so depressed, so it is better to inject between the STF and DTF. To inject at the submuscular layer, it is easier to use a needle rather than cannula, so insert the needle to the bone at the virtual circle described before. We need to consider before injection that a greater amount of filler is needed when injecting in this deepest area.

As mentioned before, the anterior 2/3 is usually depressed, but when there is posterior 1/3 depression, it is recommended to make another entry point and inject between the STF and DTF. The entry point would be 1cm above the horizontal hairline of lateral eyebrow upper margin, and this entry point would avoid nerves and vessels (Fig. 5-8).

After augmentation, if there is any irregularity or noticeable borderline, it is better to inject at the dermal and/or subdermal layer with soft fillers (Fig. 5-9).

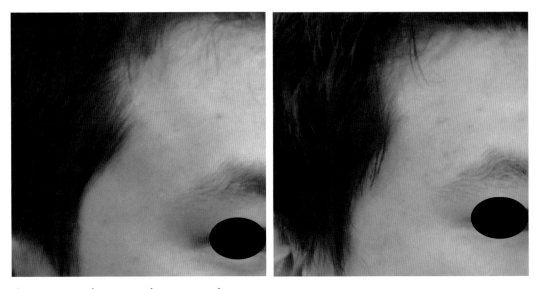

Fig. 5-9 **Pre-and post-temple augmentation**

This is a technique to observe the most depressed temporal fossa and insert the needle perpendicularly to the subperiosteal plane after avoiding the superficial temporal artery by palpation. However, the author does not recommend this technique because it might damage not just the superficial temporal artery but also the facial nerve temporal branch, middle temporal vein, and deep temporal artery and vein.

Suggestive Readings

1. Hwang K, Kim DJ. Attachment of the deep temporal fascia to the zygomatic arch: an anatomic study. The Journal of craniofacial surgery. 1999;10(4):342-5.
2. Lei T, Xu DC, Gao JH, Zhong SZ, Chen B, Yang DY, et al. Using the frontal branch of the superficial temporal artery as a landmark for locating the course of the temporal branch of the facial nerve during rhytidectomy: an anatomical study. Plastic and reconstructive surgery. 2005;116(2):623-9; discussion 30.
3. Matic DB, Kim S. Temporal hollowing following coronal incision: a prospective, randomized, controlled trial. Plastic and reconstructive surgery. 2008;121(6):379e-85e.
4. O'Brien JX, Ashton MW, Rozen WM, Ross R, Mendelson BC. New perspectives on the surgical anatomy and nomenclature of the temporal region: literature review and dissection study. Plastic and reconstructive surgery. 2013;131(3):510-22.

Temple augmentation at a glance

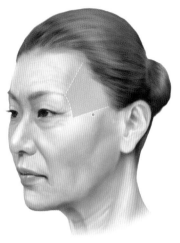
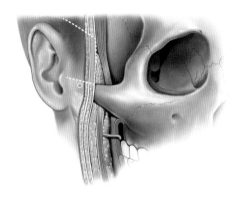

● **Dr. Hyung-Ik Baik (Plastic Surgeon)'s technique**

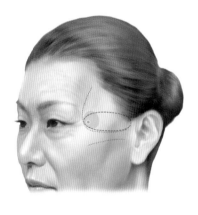
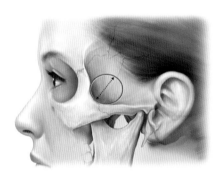

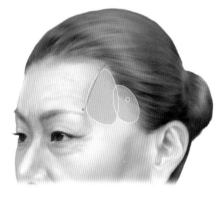
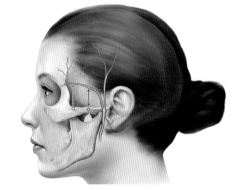

● **Dr. Gi-Woong Hong (Plastic Surgeon)'s technique**

	Dr. Baik (PS)	Dr. Hong (PS)
Needle/cannula	23G cannula	Mild depression: 23G cannula Severe depression: 21G cannula
Unilateral amount	1 mL	Mild: mid hardness 0.5~1 mL Severe: hard filler 1~1.5 mL
Elasticity The Chaeum	No.3	Mild: No.2 Severe: No.3~4
Anesthesia	Local lidocaine	EMLA cream and local anesthesia at the entry point
Techniques	Fanning technique	Mild: retrograde horizontal fanning and crossing technique Severe: fanning with sandwich technique Bolus with tower technique
Layer	STF and DTF	Mild: STF and DTF Severe: STFP or subtemporalis muscle space

CHAPTER **06**

Cheek

Anteromedial cheek

Eui-Sik Kim, M.D., Ph.D., Plastic Surgeon

6. 1. 1. 1 Design

When we discuss sunken cheek, different nomenclatures are shown in literatures. Oriental literature usually describes the buccal and lateral part, while Western literature describes the anterior part (Fig. 6-1-1).

There is a different point of view between Western and Oriental people about the location of the malar eminence to obtain the Ogee curve and/or apple cheek. Western people describe a high cheek bone as youthful oval face, usually described by Hinderer's line (line from the alar groove to tragus and line from the lateral canthus to lateral oral commissure) and superolateral part as prominent point. Oriental people tend to have wide width face and prominent zygoma, so the medial part of Hinderer's line should be prominent to have a youthful appearance (Fig. 6-1-2).

Another method is to make a patient smile naturally, and when an anteromedial protrusion is shown, augment more the area. Design and inject at a sitting position.

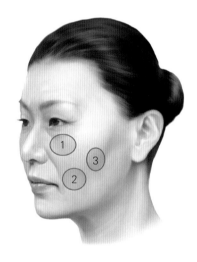

Fig. 6-1-1
Classification of cheek hollowness

1. Anteromedial(Anterior) cheek hollowness
   = Midcheek hollowness
   = Anterior maxillary depression
2. Buccal cheek hollowness (recess)
   = Sunken cheek
   = Hollow cheek
   = Submalar depression
3. Lateral cheek hollowness
   = Zygomatico-malar depression
   = Subzygoma depression

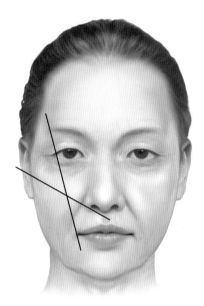

Fig. 6-1-2 **Hinderer's line**

6. 1. 1. 2 Anesthesia

Inject a small amount of lidocaine at the entry point to not disturb the desired contour.

6. 1. 1. 3 Techniques

The anatomy is as follows, from the superficial to deep layer: skin, superficial fatty layer, orbicularis oculi muscle, SOOF, deep medial cheek fat (DMCF), prezygomatic space, preperiosteal fat, and periosteum (Fig. 6-1-3). The cannula is recommended because some important structures are located here such as the inferior orbital foramen, vessel and nerve from the zygomaticofacial foramen, angular vein along the nasojugal groove, and unpredicted detoured facial artery.

The entry point would be inferolateral than the desired augmented area, which is a vertical line in the lateral canthus and horizontal line in the alar groove. This area does not relatively bruise and could avoid important structures as described above (Fig. 6-1-4).

When we augment only the superficial malar fat pad, it looks unnatural and puffy and even more when smiling, so it is better to augment the deeper layer with high-viscosity HA filler. Inject a small amount

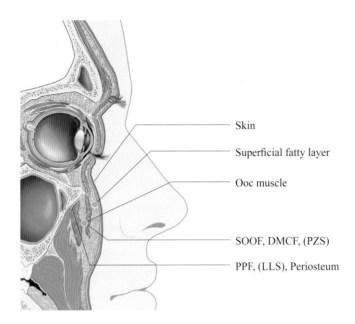

Skin

Superficial fatty layer

Ooc muscle

SOOF, DMCF, (PZS)

PPF, (LLS), Periosteum

Fig. 6-1-3 Five anatomical layers of the anteromedial cheek area

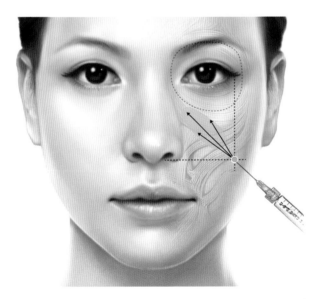

Fig. 6-1-4 Entry point for anteromedial cheek hollowness correction

into the SOOF and deep malar fat pad (DMFP), and when needed, it better to augment additionally the superficial fatty layer for a scaffold effect. The SOOF is located at the medial limbus and divides medially and laterally at the lateral canthus vertical line. The lateral SOOF is like to attach to the periosteum loosely to form a prezygomatic space. The prezygomatic space is located between the ORL upper border and zygomatico-cutaneous ligament (ZCL) lower border, and it is uncommon in Oriental people but it could be injected when there is a severe depressed zygoma. DMCF is a deep fat that is located medial to the zygomatic major muscle and located deeper than the upper lip elevators, and unlike the nasolabial fat that is superficial fat and located on the upper part, the DMCF is located on the upper and lower parts, so when volume loss starts at one part, a cascade effect of the aging process is likely to occur. The DMCF can be divided into medial and lateral by the zygomaticus major muscle and facial vein, and lateral DMCF is stuck to the bone, while the medial DMCF is attached to the bone loosely, creating Ristow's space.

The injection technique would be as follows: protect the inferior orbital rim with the non-injecting hand, insert the cannula tip, targeting SOOF and DMCF, and inject using the retrograde fanning technique. Cannula tip should not be completely out of the entry point but nearby, and insert another pathway like a windmill (Windmill technique). Overcorrection is very unnatural, so undercorrection is performed first, and minimal reinjection is recommended after 2 weeks. When correction needed multiple sites, the nasolabial fold should be corrected first. Because augmentation of the DMCF region could reduce anteromedial cheek injection, and when the anteromedial and lateral cheek area is corrected first, the face would appear much wider. Thus, the sequence would be nasolabial fold → anteromedial cheek → lateral cheek → buccal cheek.

Anteromedial cheek

Gi-Woong Hong, M.D., Ph.D., Plastic Surgeon

6. 1. 2. 1 Considerations before injection.

Regarding "sunken cheek," Oriental people tend to describe it as lateral cheek hollowness or buccal cheek hollowness, but Western people tend to describe it as anteromedial cheek (midcheek hollowness) or depressed malar eminence. Regarding "apple cheek," Western people are likely to augment the superolateral zygoma region, but since Oriental people have a prominent zygomatic arch portion, anteromedial augmentation is preferred (Fig. 6-1-5).

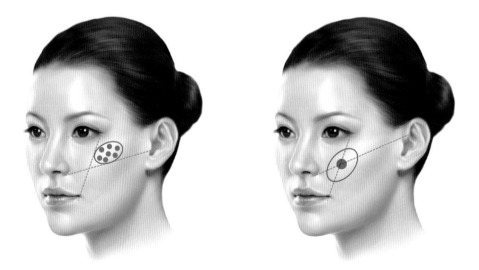

Fig. 6-1-5 **Difference of apple cheek location between Western and Oriental people**

It is recommended to augment the crossing point of the horizontal line from the alar groove upper portion to the root of the helix, tragus, and vertical line from the lateral canthus to lateral commissure of the lip. It is recommended to augment a smooth contour when smiling rather than prominent augmentation like those in Western people. The layers are as follows: skin, superficial malar fat pads, orbicularis oculi muscle, DMFPs including SOOF, mimetic muscles including zygomatic major muscle, preperiosteal fat, and periosteum. When performing an apple cheek, it is recommended to inject at the prezygomatic space where preperiosteal fat is located. When augmenting the anteromedial cheek, medial to apple cheek, it is recommended to inject DMFPs, and not to inject in bolus but spread the injection at the fatty layer. Hygiene after deep injection such as that in the anteromedial cheek is extremely important, and the patient should be warned not to apply any cosmetic products (Fig. 6-1-6).

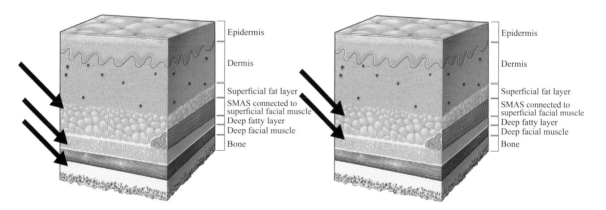

Fig. 6-1-6 **Cheeks: injection plane**

6. 1. 2. 2 Injection technique

When there is anteromedial cheek hollowness (midcheek hollowness), determine the area to augment as described previously about apple cheek, and insert either the cannula or needle, and make an entry point on the inferolateral part of the desired area. When using a needle, care should be taken to avoid the infraorbital artery, infraorbital nerve, zygomaticofacial artery, and zygomaticofacial nerve. When augmenting the medial part of the anteromedial cheek, should be taken to avoid the facial vein, which is along the nasojugal groove, and the infraorbital branch of the duplex facial artery, which can be seen in 30% of Oriental people. When using the cannula, make an entry point at the level of the vertical line from the lateral orbital rim and horizontal line from the mid-alar groove, and should avoid the above mentioned arteries (Fig. 6-1-7).

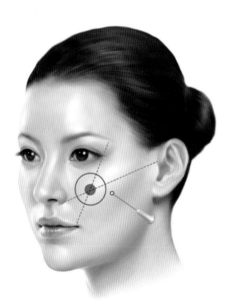

Top of apple cheek mound
- Line from lateral canthus to mouth commissure
- Line from root of helix to nasal alar base

Mid-cheek hollow injection entry point
1) Lateral and inferior to area requiring volume
2) Lateral part of mid-cheek on the vertical line of the lateral orbital rim and horizontal line of mid-alar groove

Mid-cheek hollow injection technique
1) Retrograde fanning, crossing technique
2) Vertical bolus and layering technique
- Perlane or subQ 0.7~1 mL for each area of mid-cheek hollow or mid-cheek groove : 27G or 23G cannula or needle
- Restylane lidocaine 0.3~0.5 mL each area for subdermal injection to smooth out the surface

Fig. 6-1-7 Anteromedial cheek hollow: Injection point and techniques

When there is a depressed zygomatic bone, it is recommended to augment the prezygomatic space with a hard filler, but Oriental people rarely have a depressed bony part, so it is recommended to augment DMFPs including the SOOF above the upper lip elevator muscles. The non-injecting hand is used to pinch the cheek fat pads, and using retrograde fanning, cross-hatching, or layering technique, inject the filler at the desired point first. Then, moderately augment the surrounding area, and if there are some borderline or mild irregular areas, it is recommended to inject a soft filler using the tenting technique for a smooth contour (Fig. 6-1-8).

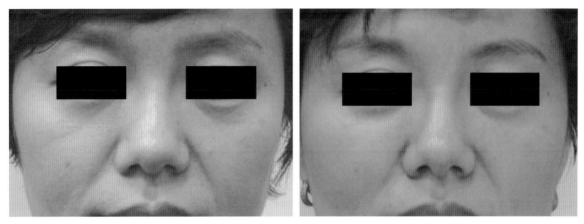

Fig. 6-1-8 Anteromedial augmentation and mid-cheek furrow: pre-and post-injection

Suggestive Readings

1. Kpodzo DS, Nahai F, McCord CD. Malar mounds and festoons: review of current management. Aesthetic surgery journal. 2014;34(2):235-48.
2. Mendelson BC, Jacobson SR. Surgical anatomy of the midcheek: facial layers, spaces, and the midcheek segments. Clinics in plastic surgery. 2008;35(3):395-404; discussion 393.
3. Mendelson BC, Muzaffar AR, Adams WP, Jr. Surgical anatomy of the midcheek and malar mounds. Plastic and reconstructive surgery. 2002;110(3):885-96; discussion 97-911.
4. Rohrich RJ, Pessa JE, Ristow B. The youthful cheek and the deep medial fat compartment. Plastic and reconstructive surgery. 2008;121(6):2107-12.

Anteromedial cheek

Hyun-Jo Kim, M.D., M.S., Dermatologist

6. 1. 3. 1 Design

The area medial to the zygomatic bone, lateral to the nasal dorsum, and above the nasolabial fold is called the anterior malar area, but as this is not an anatomical nomenclature, anteromedial cheeks is more appropriate term (Fig. 6-1-9).

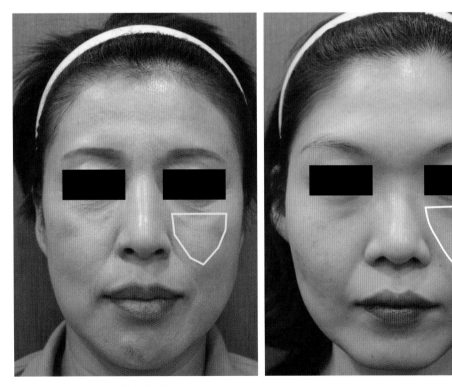

Fig. 6-1-9 **Anteromedial cheeks**

6. 1. 3. 2 Anesthesia

Filler that contains lidocaine is less painful, so EMLA cream is sufficient, but for patient's convenience, EMLA cream application and regional anesthesia, which is an infraorbital nerve block, are performed. Inform the patient to be careful about oral burn due to hot drinks or food for 3 h after infraorbital nerve block.

6. 1. 3. 3 Techniques

6. 1. 3. 3. 1 Needle versus blunt tip microcannula

The authors prefer the microcannula to minimize vascular compromise.

The entry point is made relative to the avascular point between the infraorbital and zygomaticofacial arteries (Fig. 6-1-10). Puncture using a 23G needle, insert a 23G blunt-tip microcannula at the periosteum

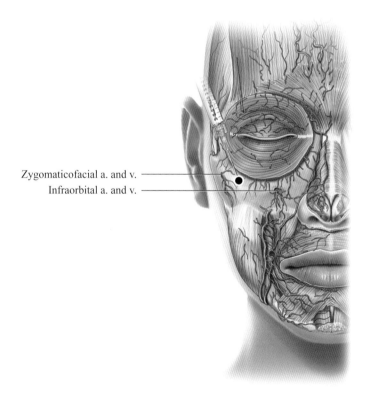

Zygomaticofacial a. and v.
Infraorbital a. and v.

Fig. 6-1-10 Anteromedial cheeks injection entry points

level, and inject the filler as shown in Fig. 6-1-11.

6. 1. 3. 3. 2 Filler amount

There is a different volume needed for each person, but an average of 1~2 mL of filler is injected unilaterally.

6. 1. 3. 3. 3 Progress and photograph

A case of anteromedial cheek augmentation and correction of tear trough deformity (Fig. 6-1-12).

A case of anteromedial cheek augmentation and nasolabial fold correction, forehead augmentation, and chin augmentation (Fig. 6-1-13).

Midface aging phenomenon is not a solitary change but has an intimate relationship between facial areas, so patient's satisfaction also increases when these aging signs are corrected.

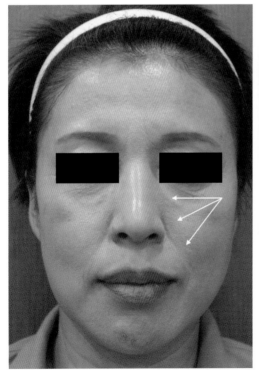

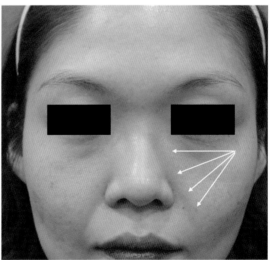

Fig. 6-1-11
Anteromedial cheek filler injection technique by cannula

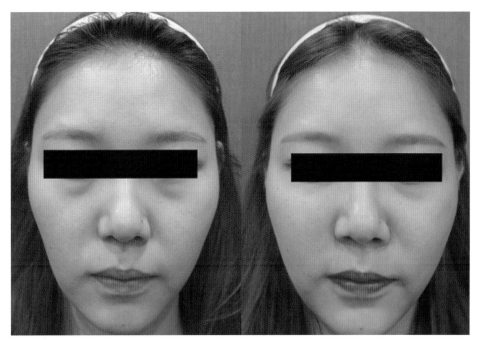

Fig. 6-1-12 **Tear trough deformity and anteromedial cheek filler injection: before and after**

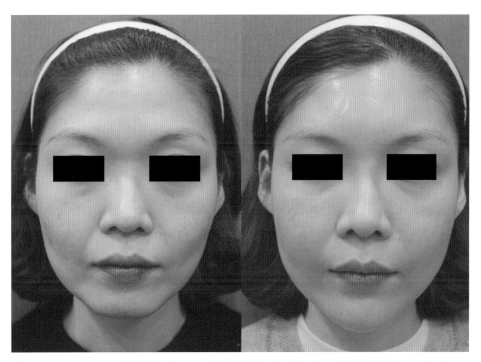

Fig. 6-1-13 **Anteromedial cheeks, nasolabial folds, forehead, and chin: before and after**

6. 1. 3. 3. 4 Cautions

Care should be taken to avoid the infraorbital trunk type, detoured branch (Fig. 6-1-14) because it is not a traditional branch and runs through the anteromedial cheek area. The infraorbital trunk usually runs at the subcutaneous layer, so it is relatively safe to approach below the muscles, such as the periosteum layer and use a blunt-tip microcannula.

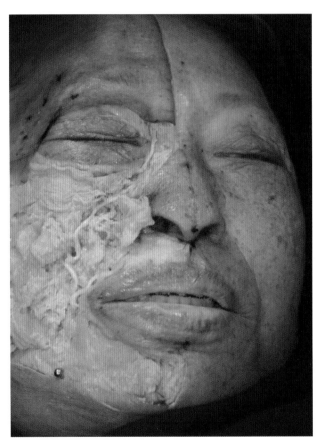

Fig. 6-1-14 **Detoured Branch of Facial Artery**

Suggestive Readings

1. Kim H-J, Seo KK, Lee H-K, Kim J. Clinical Anatomy of the Face for Filler and Botulinum Toxin Injection: Springer; 2016.
2. Wong CH, Mendelson B. Newer Understanding of Specific Anatomic Targets in the Aging Face as Applied to Injectables: Aging Changes in the Craniofacial Skeleton and Facial Ligaments. Plastic and reconstructive surgery. 2015;136(5 Suppl):44s-8s.
3. Yang HM, Lee JG, Hu KS, Gil YC, Choi YJ, Lee HK, et al. New anatomical insights on the course and branching patterns of the facial artery: clinical implications of injectable treatments to the nasolabial fold and nasojugal groove. Plastic and reconstructive surgery. 2014;133(5):1077-82.

Anteromedial cheek techniques at a glance

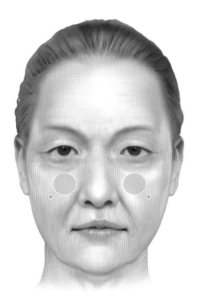
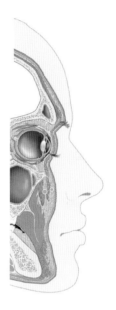

• Dr. Eui-Sik Kim (Plastic Surgeon)'s technique

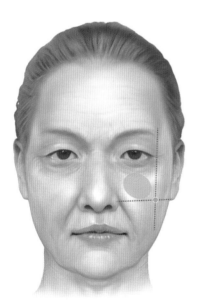
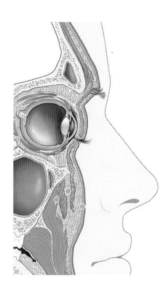

• Dr. Gi-Woong Hong (Plastic Surgeon)'s technique

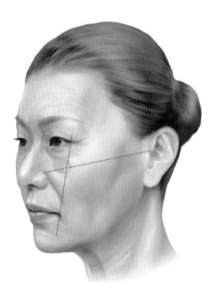 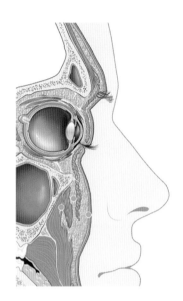

• **Dr. Gi-Woong Hong (Plastic Surgeon)'s technique**

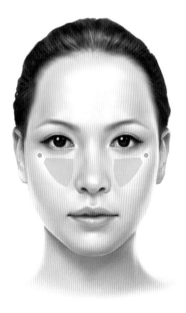 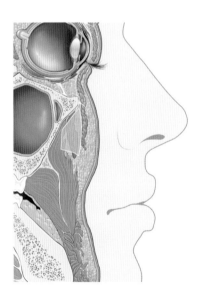

• **Dr. Hyun-Jo Kim (Dermatologist)'s technique**

	Dr. Kim ES (PS)	Dr. Hong (PS)	Dr. Kim HJ (Derma)
Needle/cannula	23G cannula	Deep: 21G cannula or 23G needle Superficial: 30G needle	23G cannula
Unilateral amount	0.5~1 mL	1~1.5 mL	1.5~2 mL
Elasticity The Chaeum	Superficial: No.2 Deep: No.3	Hard: No.3 or No.4 Soft: No.1 or No.2	No.2
Anesthesia	EMLA cream and entry point lidocaine	Cannula: EMLA cream & entry point lidocaine Needle: EMLA cream	Regional nerve block and EMLA cream
Techniques	Retrograde fanning	Deep: retrograde fanning and crossing technique and vertical bolus and layering technique Superficial: linear threading and droplet injection and tenting technique	Modified fan technique: windmill technique
Layer	Layer 2 (subcutaneous) Severe: layer 4 (SOOF, DMCF)	Deep: SOOF and DMCF, prezygomatic space Superficial: subdermal and superficial subcutaneous layer	Periosteum or submuscular layer

Buccal cheek

Hyun-Jo Kim, M.D., M.S., Dermatologist

6. 2. 1. 1 Design

Buccal fat pads support superficial fat with DMCF. Sunken cheek is caused by decreased volume and descent of buccal fat and usually creates an aging appearance.

Deep medial cheek fat covers the upper cheek above the nasolabial fold, and buccal fat pad covers volumes of the region between the mouth angle and masseter muscle (Fig. 6-2-1).

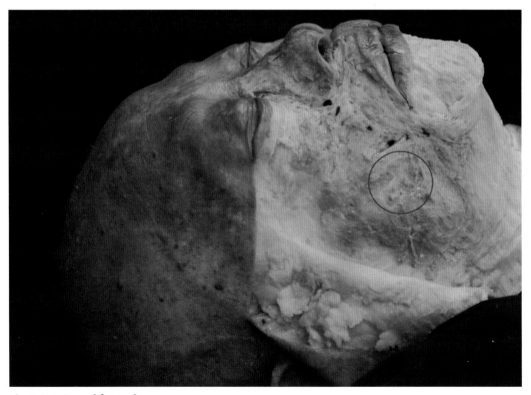

Fig. 6-2-1 **Buccal fat pad**

6. 2. 1. 2 Anesthesia

EMLA cream application is enough when a filler containing lidocaine is used.

6. 2. 1. 3 Techniques

6. 2. 1. 3. 1 Needle or blunt-tip cannula

Both methods are available. The author prefers to use the needle, perforating perpendicularly the most depressed area and injecting into the deepest layer of buccal fat first and then superficial fat layer using the tower technique.

6. 2. 1. 3. 2 Filler amount

A relatively large volume is needed to inject in the deep and superficial fat. Unilateral injection of 2~4 mL of filler is performed.

6. 2. 1. 3. 3 Progress and photograph

Correction of sunken cheek by injection in the deep and superficial fat at the buccal fat area (Fig. 6-2-2).

6. 2. 1. 3. 4 Cautions

The parotid duct tends to run from the tragus to mouth angle, so it is recommended to mark the location and not to make an entry point. Usually, the facial artery does not run through it, but there would be variations, so always be careful to avoid vascular compromise.

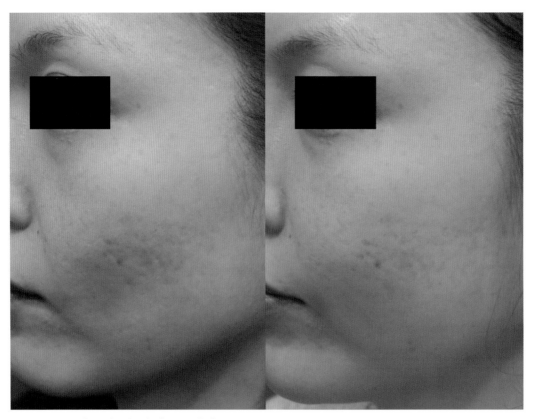

Fig. 6-2-2 **Sunken cheeks: before and after**

Suggestive Readings

1. Gierloff M, Stohring C, Buder T, Gassling V, Acil Y, Wiltfang J. Aging changes of the midfacial fat compartments: a computed tomographic study. Plastic and reconstructive surgery. 2012;129(1):263-73.
2. Rohrich RJ, Pessa JE. The anatomy and clinical implications of perioral submuscular fat. Plastic and reconstructive surgery. 2009;124(1):266-71.

Choon-ShikYoun, M.D., Dermatologist

6. 2. 2. 1 Pathophysiology

6. 2. 2. 1. 1 Reduced volume and descent of superficial fat and deep fat

Buccal area volume loss occurs by volume loss and descent migration of superficial and deep fat (buccal fat).

6. 2. 2. 1. 2 Bone resorption

Buccal area volume loss is aggravated by soft tissue supporting structure, zygoma, and maxillary bone resorption.

6. 2. 2. 1. 3 Retaining tissue loosening

Buccal area volume loss is aggravated by loosening of retaining tissue of the skin, fat, and muscle.

6. 2. 2. 2 Design and surface anatomy

The buccal cheek is located between the malar (zygomatic angle) and jowl fat and indicates buccal fat and anterior part of the modiolus anatomically (Fig. 6-2-3).

6. 2. 2. 3 Anesthesia

6. 2. 2. 3. 1 EMLA cream application

The buccal region is relatively less painful, and EMLA cream application would be adequate. The author just applies EMLA cream when filler injection is through a needle.

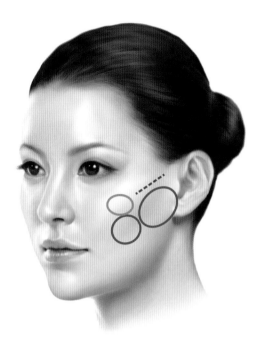

Fig. 6-2-3 **Buccal cheek: surface anatomy**

6. 2. 2. 3. 2 Local anesthesia lidocaine injection

Pain can occur during treatment and postinjection. Postinjection pain is reduced by injecting lidocaine. The author prefers to inject lidocaine when a cannula is used.

6. 2. 2. 4 Techniques

6. 2. 2. 4. 1 Needle

Usually, the target layer is the subcutaneous layer (layer 2), and the target fat is the medial cheek fat (Fig. 6-2-4). Usually, design the contour line and inject in the deepest part using the vertical injection technique 1cm apart.

Inject 0.4 mL at deeply sunken and 0.1 mL at superficially sunken area, depending on the point depth (Fig. 6-2-5).

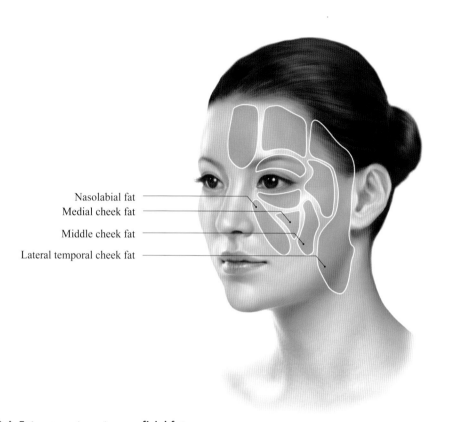

Nasolabial fat
Medial cheek fat
Middle cheek fat
Lateral temporal cheek fat

Fig. 6-2-4 **Fat compartment: superficial fat**

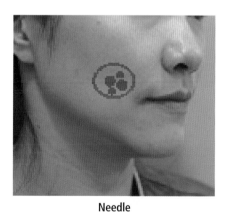

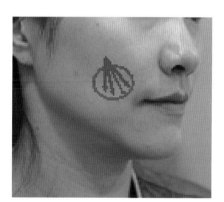

Needle

Cannula

Fig. 6-2-5 **Design & Injection technique**

Injection depth would be on the deep part of the fat layer, and for minimal correction, inject at the superficial fat layer (Fig. 6-2-6).

* The anatomical location in the buccal area is anterior to the masseter muscle and below the maxilla and zygoma.

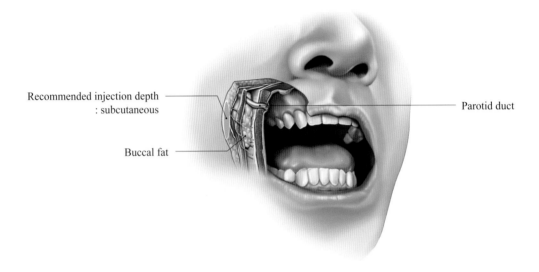

Recommended injection depth
: subcutaneous

Buccal fat

Parotid duct

Fig. 6-2-6 Injection depth

6. 2. 2. 4. 2 Cannula

Usually, inject targeting the subcutaneous layer. Make an entry point above the drawn contour line, and inject the filler at the deepest part using the linear threading technique and at the surrounding area using the fan technique (Fig. 6-2-5).

Injection depth would be the deep part of the fatty layer, and avoid irregularity by injecting the filler evenly (Fig. 6-2-6).

6. 2. 2. 5 Filler amount

The amount depends on the depth and size of the layer, and an average of 0.5~1.5 mL is injected on each side.

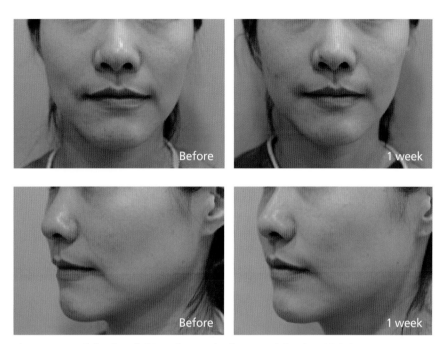

Fig. 6-2-7 Preinjection (left) and 1 week after postinjection (right)
Buccal cheek: Belotero volume, 1 mL/side, cannula

6. 2. 2. 6 Progress and photograph

6. 2. 2. 6. 1 Buccal cheek filler preinjection and postinjection (Fig. 6-2-7)

6. 2. 2. 6. 2 Buccal and lateral cheek filler injection

Buccal cheek depression is likely to combine with lateral cheek depression, and in this case, the lateral cheek also has to be augmented for better results. The facial contour line is smoother when the lateral cheek is simultaneously corrected (Fig. 6-2-8).

6. 2. 2. 7 Cautions

There are few fibrotic bands between the skin and SMAS layer. However, when the filler is injected at buccal the fat pad under the SMAS layer, there might be some problems: (1) aggravation of buccal fat descent and jowl or Marionette's line, (2) damage to the parotid duct and facial nerve (Fig. 6-2-9), and (3) increase in the amount of needed filler compared to that injected at layer 2 (subcutaneous).

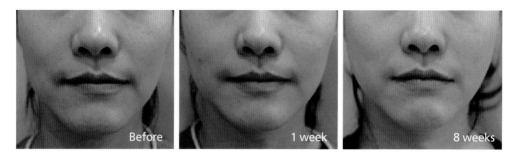

Fig. 6-2-8 Preinjection view, 1 week after buccal cheek injection, 8 weeks after buccal cheek injection, and 7 weeks after lateral cheek injection

Buccal cheek: Belotero volume, 1 mL/side, cannula, Lateral cheek: Belotero volume, 1 mL/side, cannula

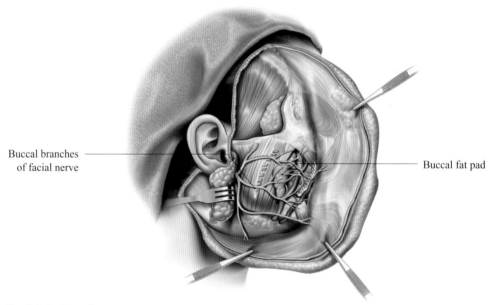

Buccal branches
of facial nerve

Buccal fat pad

Fig. 6-2-9 Buccal space

Eui-Sik Kim, M.D., Ph.D., Plastic Surgeon

6. 2. 3. 1 Design

Generally, the "sunken cheek" usually means the area that is anterior to masseter muscle and below maxilla and zygoma is sunken. Traditionally, Oriental people thought rounded cheeks appears young looking, so cheek hollowness result in gaunt, poor, and even depressed look. In the aging process, reduced volume of buccal fat, descent, and prominent hollowness are observed. Since the depressed area and amount are different in the sitting and supine positions, design and injection should be performed in the sitting position.

6. 2. 3. 2 Anesthesia

Inject a small amount of lidocaine at the entry point to not disturb the desired contour.

6. 2. 3. 3 Techniques

The buccal cheek layers are as follows: skin → superficial fat layer → mimetic muscle and SMAS → buccal fat → buccinator → oral mucosa. Unlike those in other regions, all structures are supported by soft tissue and not by bone (Fig. 6-2-10).

Injection point will be under the sunken area, and pulsation of the facial artery should be felt at the winding portion, which is located superolateral from the modiolus, and this vessel should be avoid unless there would be severe bleeding and bruising (Fig. 6-2-11).

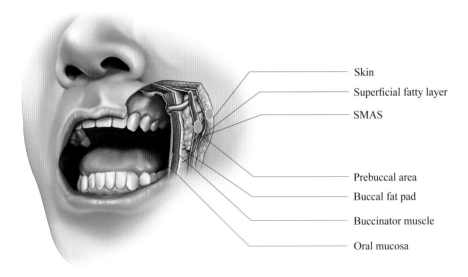

Skin
Superficial fatty layer
SMAS

Prebuccal area
Buccal fat pad
Buccinator muscle
Oral mucosa

Fig. 6-2-10 Five anatomical layers of the buccal cheek area

When there is a mild sunken area, inject an adequate amount of filler at the subcutaneous fat layer using retrograde fanning technique by either a needle or cannula. If the area is severely sunken, consider a dual-plane injection. Since the cannula tip is not noticeable when located deeply, locate the cannula tip at the prebuccal area above the buccal capsule (fascia), and inject the hard filler with the same method as to injecting at the bony area first. Then, inject at the second subcutaneous layer, and finally inject a soft filler at the subdermal layer.

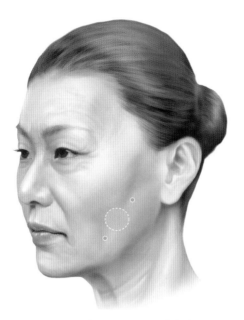

Fig. 6-2-11 Entry point for buccal cheek hollowness correction

Buccal fat is located in the triangular area of the zygomaticus major and risorius muscles, and buccal cheek hollowness occur during the aging process. Thus, in view of the cause, the filler should be injected in the buccal fat, but it is not recommended due to the following reasons. First, volumizing buccal fat causes not only surface augmentation but also mucosal hypertrophy. Second, jowl ptosis is aggravated due to gravitational descent. Third, the parotid duct and facial nerve are located at the buccal fat. Lastly, a large amount of filler is needed.

It is recommended to augment the anteriomedial cheek before the buccal cheek. When this area is overcorrected, the results would be aesthetically unsatisfactory because of a round face.

Buccal cheek

Gi-Woong Hong, M.D., Ph.D., Plastic Surgeon

6. 2. 4. 1 Considerations before injection

The buccal area layers are as follows: skin, subcutaneous layer, mimetic muscles and SMAS, buccal fat pad, deep muscle layer, and oral mucosa. The recommended injection layers are the subcutaneous layer and undersurface of the SMAS. In injecting at the buccal fat pad, a large amount of filler is needed, and descent ptosis might develop because of loose connective tissues.

6. 2. 4. 2 Techniques

First, design the buccal cheek hollowness, and make an entry point beneath the desired area. Then, augment using retrograde fanning technique or cross-hatching technique by a needle or cannula. Subse-

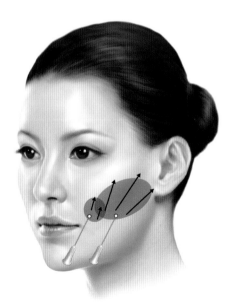

Buccal and lateral cheek hollow injection entry point for superficial injection
- Inferior to buccal and submalar area for superficial fat injection

Buccal and lateral cheek hollow injection technique
 • Retrograde horizontal fanning
- Perlane 0.7~1 mL for superficial fat injection
: 27G cannula or nano needle
   - Restylane lidocaine 0.3~0.5 mL each area for subdermal injection to smooth out the surface

Fig. 6-2-12 Mild buccal cheek hollow: Injection point and techniques

quently, inject the subdermal layer with a soft filler to make smooth contour (Fig. 6-2-12).

When the area is severely depressed, a cannula is recommended because the area is deeper than the SMAS and care should be taken to avoid the vessel and facial nerve. The recommended puncture site is 4 cm anterior from the tragus and 2 cm below the inferior border of the zygomatic arch. After perforating the hard tissue of the SMAS layer, the prebuccal space could be felt, which is outside the buccal fat pad capsule. Thus, it is better to inject this layer first and then the subcutaneous layer for smooth contour.

Suggestive Readings

1. Pessa JE, Rohrich RJ. Facial Topography: Clinical Anatomy of the Face: Quality Medical Pub.; 2012.
2. Rohrich RJ, Pessa JE. The fat compartments of the face: anatomy and clinical implications for cosmetic surgery. Plastic and reconstructive surgery. 2007;119(7):2219-27; discussion 28-31.
3. Yousuf S, Tubbs RS, Wartmann CT, Kapos T, Cohen-Gadol AA, Loukas M. A review of the gross anatomy, functions, pathology, and clinical uses of the buccal fat pad. Surgical and radiologic anatomy : SRA. 2010;32(5):427-36.
4. Zhang HM, Yan YP, Qi KM, Wang JQ, Liu ZF. Anatomical structure of the buccal fat pad and its clinical adaptations. Plastic and reconstructive surgery. 2002;109(7):2509-18; discussion 19-20.

Buccal cheek augmentation at a glance

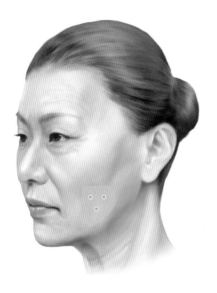

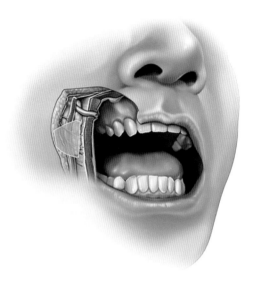

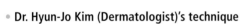

● **Dr. Hyun-Jo Kim (Dermatologist)'s technique**

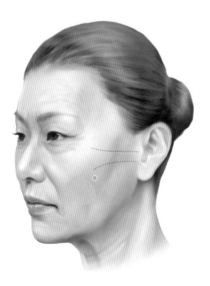

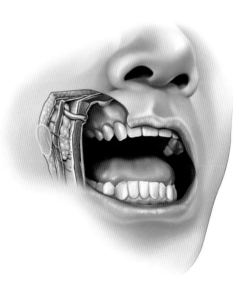

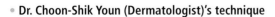

● **Dr. Choon-Shik Youn (Dermatologist)'s technique**

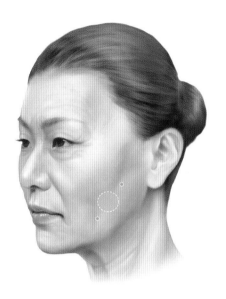

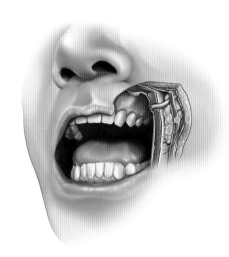

• **Dr. Eui-Sik Kim (Plastic Surgeon)'s technique**

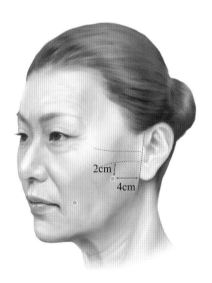

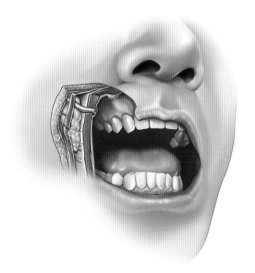

• **Dr. Gi-Woong Hong (Plastic Surgeon)'s technique**

	Dr. Kim HJ (Derma)	Dr. Youn (Derma)	Dr. Kim ES (PS)	Dr. Hong (PS)
Needle/cannula	27G 13 mm needle	23G cannula	23G cannula	Severe: 23G cannula Mild depression: 30G needle
Unilateral amount	2~3 mL	0.5~1.5 mL	0.5~1.5 mL	Severe depression: hard filler 0.7~1 mL Mild depression: soft filler 0.3~0.5 mL
Elasticity The Chaeum	No.2 or 3	No.4	Superficial: No.2 Deep: No.3	Hard: No.3 Soft: No.2
Anesthesia	EMLA cream	EMLA cream	EMLA cream and entry point local lidocaine	EMLA cream and entry point local lidocaine
Techniques	Tower technique (bolus injection)	Fanning + linear threading technique	Retrograde fanning	Severe: retrograde fanning and crossing, layering techniques Mild: linear threading and fanning technique
Layer	Deep fat (layer 4) Superficial fat (layer2)	Subcutaneous	Layer 2 + layer 4 (prebuccal area) + buccal fat	Severe: prebuccal space Mild: subcutaneous

Hyun-Jo Kim, M.D., M.S., Dermatologist

6. 3. 1. 1 Design

Below the zygomatic arch, submalar area volume loss results in an aging appearance. Draw a contour line at the depressed area.

6. 3. 1. 2 Anesthesia

A filler that contains lidocaine is less painful, so the EMLA cream is sufficient, but for patient's convenience, EMLA cream application and local lidocaine injection at the entry point are performed.

6. 3. 1. 3 Techniques

6. 3. 1. 3. 1 Needle versus blunt-tip microcannula

Both methods are available. The author prefers to use a blunt-tip microcannula because it is unnecessary to inject in the deep fat, and volume restoration is adequate when injecting at the superficial fat compartment, which is the lateral temporal cheek fat. The entry point would be the vertical line from the lateral canthus and slightly below the horizontal line from the ala nasi, and inject using the fanning technique (Fig. 6-3-1).

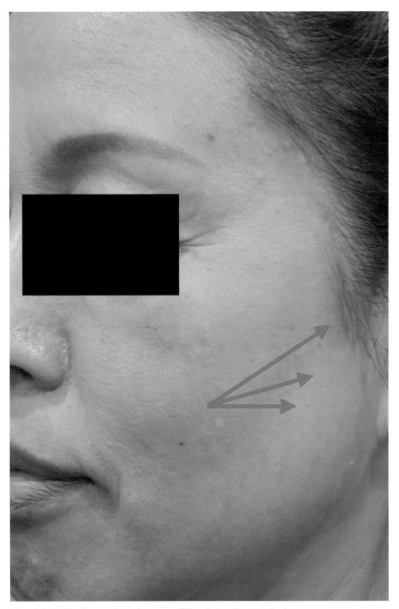

Fig. 6-3-1 Sunken submalar area filler injection technique

6. 3. 1. 3. 2 Filler amount

Unilateral injection of 1~2 mL is adequate because it is effective to augment just the superficial fat compartment.

6. 3. 1. 3. 3 Progress and photograph

Filler is injected at the sunken submalar area (Fig. 6-3-2).

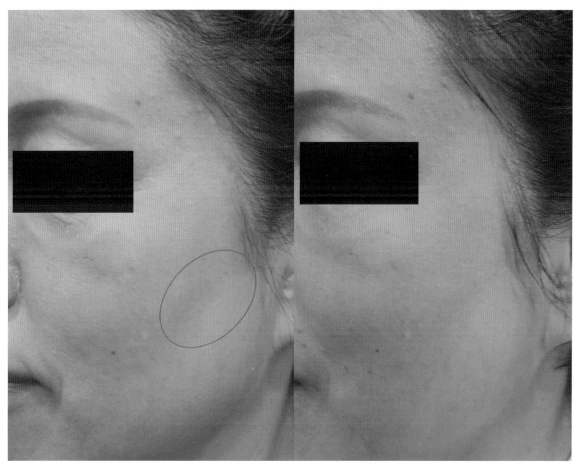

Fig. 6-3-2 **Sunken submalar area filler injection, before and after**

6. 3. 1. 3. 4 Cautions

An entry point near the tragus could be made, but superficial temporal artery damage should be considered. The transverse facial artery runs in this area, so it is better to find the pulsation to avoid vascular compromise (Fig. 6-3-3).

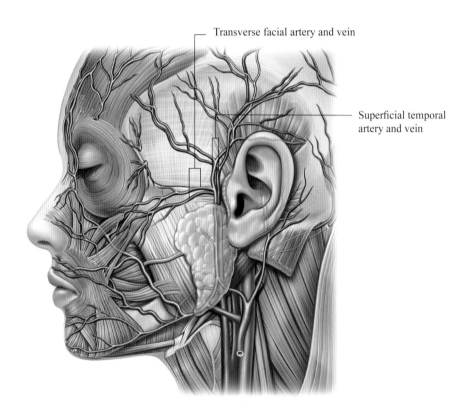

Transverse facial artery and vein

Superficial temporal artery and vein

Fig. 6-3-3 Cautious vessel of sunken submalar area filler injection

Suggestive Readings

1. Rohrich RJ, Pessa JE. The fat compartments of the face: anatomy and clinical implications for cosmetic surgery. Plastic and reconstructive surgery. 2007;119(7):2219-27; discussion 28-31.
2. Wan D, Amirlak B, Rohrich R, Davis K. The clinical importance of the fat compartments in midfacial aging. Plastic and reconstructive surgery Global open. 2013;1(9):e92.

Lateral cheek

Choon-Shik Youn, M.D., Dermatologist

6. 3. 2. 1 Pathophysiology

Buccal fat volume reduction and descent migration lead to volume loss below the zygomatic arch area. It develops by masseter muscle and superficial fat volume reduction and descent migration.

6. 3. 2. 2 Design and surface anatomy

It is located between the zygomatic arch and upper border of lower face and consists of the parotid gland and some mastication muscles (Fig. 6-3-4).

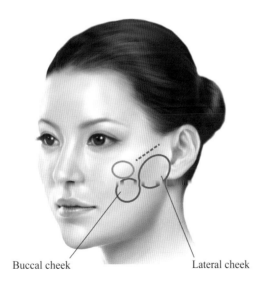

Buccal cheek   Lateral cheek

Fig. 6-3-4 **Design and surface anatomy of the lateral cheek**

6. 3. 2. 3 Anesthesia

6. 3. 2. 3. 1 EMLA cream application

This area is relatively painful, but since there are many fillers, including lidocaine, EMLA cream application might be adequate.

6. 3. 2. 3. 2 Lidocaine injection

Pain can occur during treatment and postinjection. Postinjection pain is reduced by injecting lidocaine. The author prefers to inject lidocaine when using a cannula.

6. 3. 2. 4 Techniques

6. 3. 2. 4. 1 Needle or cannula

Needle:

The target layer is the subcutaneous layer (layer 2), which is the middle cheek fat and lateral temporal cheek fat (Fig. 6-3-5). Usually, inject into the deepest portion of the sunken area using vertical injection technique 1cm apart. Usually, when the sunken area is deep, 0.4 mL of filler is injected, but when it is shallow, 0.1mL of filler is injected. Inject at the deep and superficial portions of the subcutaneous fat layer (Fig. 6-3-6).

Cannula:

The target layer is the subcutaneous layer. Design at contour line, and make an entry point above it. Inject using the linear threading technique at the deep portion, and then inject in the surrounding area using the fan technique (Fig. 6-3-6).

* In the author's personal experience, the needle has advantages of more precise filling and more volumization by small amount, while the cannula has advantages of less risk of bruising and swelling and even distribution of filler injection. Thus, when the patient has a thin skin and needs quick recovery time, the author prefers to use a cannula, and when the patient has a thick skin and does not bother about the recovery time, the author chooses a needle.

120

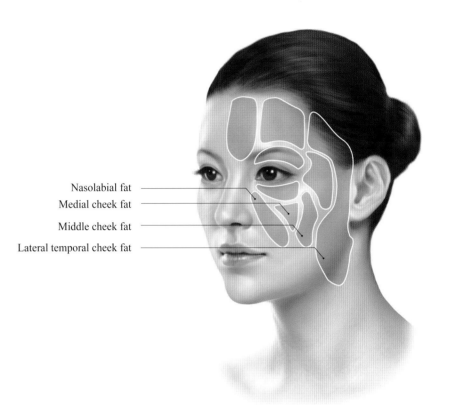

Nasolabial fat
Medial cheek fat
Middle cheek fat
Lateral temporal cheek fat

Fig. 6-3-5 **Fat compartments**

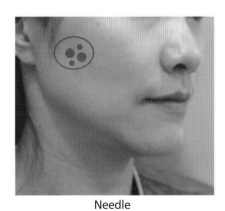

Needle

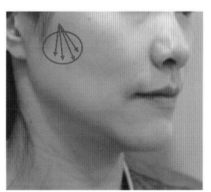

Cannula

Fig. 6-3-6 **Techniques**

* Lateral cheek depression is located at the posterior masseter muscle under the zygomatic arch. The lateral cheek has compact fibrotic bands, so high resistance would be felt and there is a high risk of uneven injection.

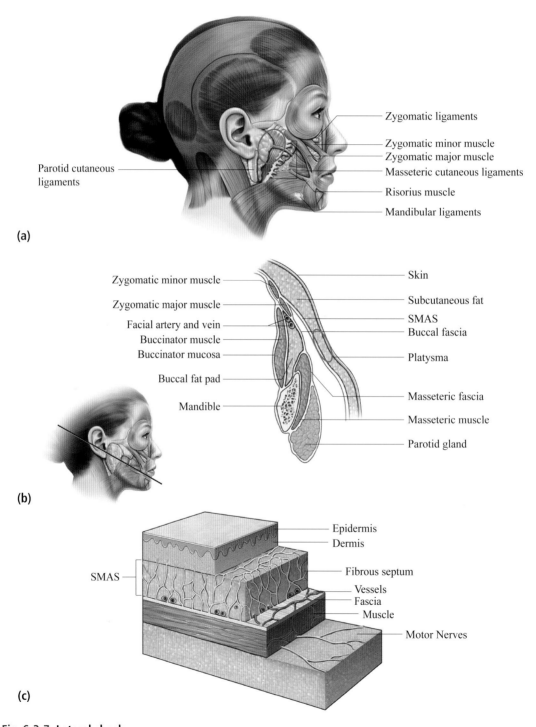

Fig. 6-3-7 Lateral cheek

6. 3. 2. 4. 2 Filler amount

The filler amount depends on the depth, but the average if 1~2 mL on each side (Fig. 6-3-8).

Depression depth: volume

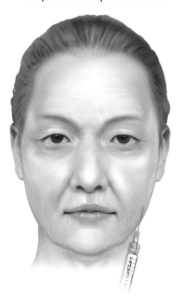

Depression Depth :
Slight depression
0.5 mL

Medium depression
0.5~1.5 mL

Deep depression
1.5~2.5 mL

Fig. 6-3-8 Injection volume

6. 3. 2. 5 Progress and photograph

Three days after filler injection, the right lateral cheek, which was injected using a cannula, had minimal swelling and no bruising, but the left lateral cheek, which was injected using a needle, had swelling and bruising (Fig. 6-3-9).

Cannula   Needle

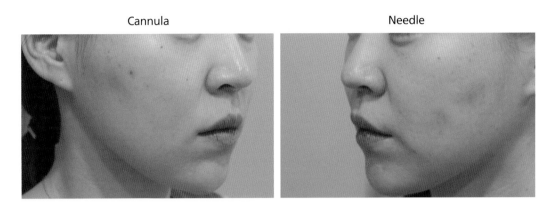

Fig. 6-3-9 Comparison between cannula and needle injection, three days after injection

Volumization effect is better at the left lateral cheek, which was injected using a needle, than at the right lateral cheek, which was injected using a cannula (Fig. 6-3-10).

Cannula   Needle

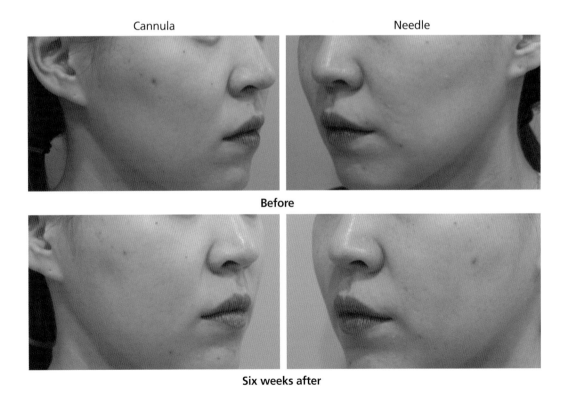

Before

Six weeks after

Fig. 6-3-10 Subjective satisfaction (volume effect)

A case of simultaneous correction of the lateral cheek, buccal cheek, and perioral chin could create a V line shape when performed simultaneously (Fig. 6-3-11).

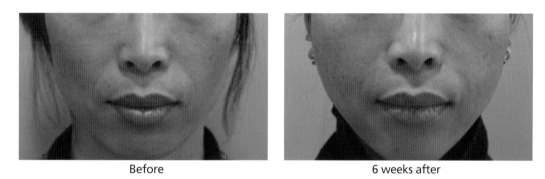

Before   6 weeks after

Fig. 6-3-11 Before and 6 weeks after filler injection

Lateral cheek: Elravie deepline 2.1 mL/side, buccal cheek: Elravie deepline 1.4 mL/side,
Nasolabial fold: Belotero balance 1.1 mL/side, chin: Elravie deepline 1 mL

Fourteen months after filler injection, volume was still maintained compared to that 6 weeks after injection, by photograph (Fig. 6-3-12).

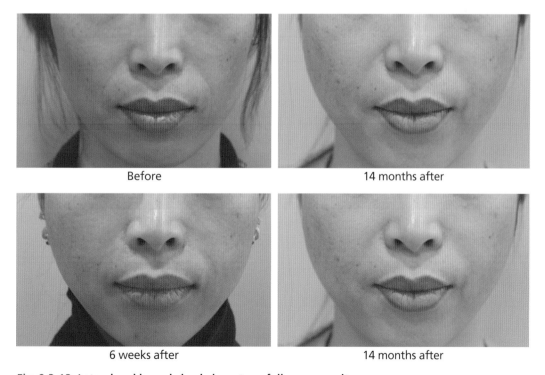

Before   14 months after

6 weeks after   14 months after

Fig. 6-3-12 Lateral and buccal cheek: long-term follow-up results

Preinjection/14 months after/6 weeks after/14 months after

A case of simultaneous correction of the buccal cheek and anteromedial cheek. Correction of the sunken area would make the face smaller and lifted (Fig. 6-3-13).

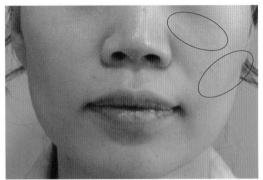

Before

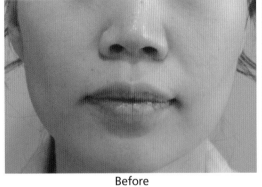

Before   9 weeks after

Fig. 6-3-13 Before and 9 weeks after filler injection

Lateral cheek: Elravie deepline 1.1 mL/side
Buccal cheek: Elravie deepline 2 mL/side
Tear trough and anteromedial cheek: Elravie deepline 1.4 mL/side = total 9 mL

Forty months after injection, the volume was still maintained compared to that 6 weeks after injection, by photograph (Fig. 6-3-14).

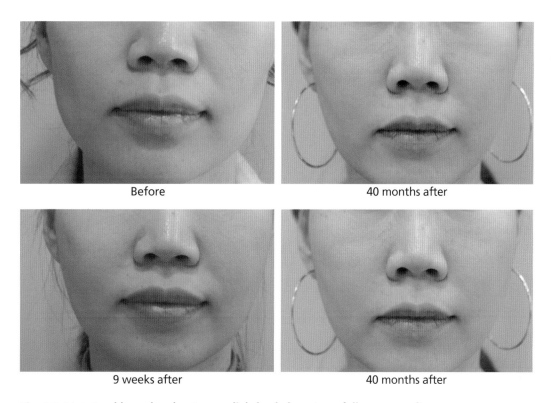

| Before | 40 months after |
| 9 weeks after | 40 months after |

Fig. 6-3-14 **Lateral buccal and anteromedial cheek: long-term follow-up results**

6. 3. 2. 6 Cautions

There are many fibrotic bands between the skin and SMAS layer at the lateral cheek, so the injected filler might migrate into the surrounding tissues when the injected area overcomes limitations. Thus, when elevation stops during injection, it is better to stop and correct the superficial layer after 6~8 weeks (Fig. 6-3-15).

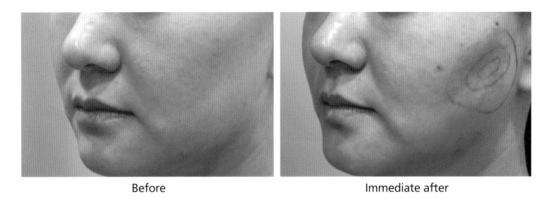

Before   Immediate after

Fig. 6-3-15 Doughnut phenomena

When injecting in the subSMAS (layer 4), avoid the parotid duct and facial nerve (Fig. 6-3-16).

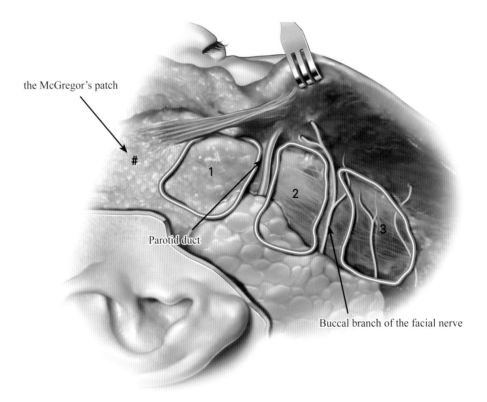

Fig. 6-3-16 Dissection is performed in layer 4

between the SMAS (uplifted) and the deep fascia (parotid masseteric fascia) The superior (1) middle (2) and the inferior (3) premasseter compartments are encircled.

CHAPTER
6-3
/3

Gi-Woong Hong, M.D., Ph.D., Plastic Surgeon

6. 3. 3. 1 Considerations before injection

When there is depression below the zygomatic arch, it is likely to be corrected because of a prominent zygoma and irregular facial contour. However, when there is severe depression or developed ZCL, which originates from the zygomatic arch inferior border to the skin, it is likely not to be elevated after filler injection, and the filler might spread to the surrounding area. Thus, in this case, undermining by the cannula should be performed and spaces should be made for filler injection.

6. 3. 3. 2 Techniques

When there is mild depression, design the borderline of injection area, and then augment from the lower to upper part at the subcutaneous layer using a needle or cannula. When there is irregular contour, inject a soft filler in the subdermal layer. When an entry point for undermining is needed, make an entry point at the crossing point of the vertical line from the lateral orbital rim margin and line from the oral commissure to tragus. Release some fibers and then inject at the deep fat, which is between the SMAS and parotid-masseteric fascia by retrograde fanning and layering technique. Then, inject a soft filler at the subdermal layer (Fig. 6-3-17).

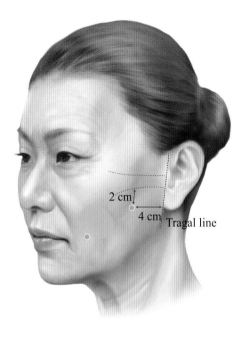

Buccal and lateral cheek hollow injection entry point for deep injection
- 4 cm anterior to tragal line and 2 cm below from lower margin of the zygomatic arch for deeper injection (subSMAS layer)
- cross of the line from the mouth commissure to tragus and the vertical line of lateral orbital rim for subSMAS layer or buccal fat pad

Buccal and lateral cheek hollow injection technique
• Retrograde horizontal fanning
- SubQ 0.7~1 mL for deep layer injection
  : 23G cannula
- Restylane lidocaine 0.3~0.5 mL each area for subdermal injection to smooth out the surface

Fig. 6-3-17 Lateral cheek hollow: injection point and techniques

Suggestive Readings

1. Cohen JL, Brown MR. Anatomic considerations for soft tissue augmentation of the face. Journal of drugs in dermatology : JDD. 2009;8(1):13-6.
2. Mendelson BC, Wong CH. Surgical anatomy of the middle premasseter space and its application in sub-SMAS face lift surgery. Plastic and reconstructive surgery. 2013;132(1):57-64.
3. Nakajima H, Imanishi N, Minabe T, Kishi K, Aiso S. Anatomical study of subcutaneous adipofascial tissue: a concept of the protective adipofascial system (PAFS) and lubricant adipofascial system (LAFS). Scandinavian journal of plastic and reconstructive surgery and hand surgery. 2004;38(5):261-6.
4. Pilsl U, Anderhuber F, Rzany B. Anatomy of the cheek: implications for soft tissue augmentation. Dermatologic surgery : official publication for American Society for Dermatologic Surgery [et al]. 2012;38(7 Pt 2):1254-62.

Eui-Sik Kim, M.D., Ph.D., Plastic Surgeon

6. 3. 4. 1 Design

Women like to correct lateral cheek hollowness under the zygomatic arch because a prominent zygoma looks masculine. During the aging process, the masseteric cutaneous ligament which is a false retaining ligament located anterior to the masseter muscle, is likely to lose supporting ability and develops SMAS loosening and skin ptosis. Design and inject at the sitting position.

6. 3. 4. 2 Anesthesia

Inject a small amount of lidocaine at the entry point to not disturb the desired contour.

6. 3. 4. 3 Techniques

The layers are as follows: skin → subcutaneous fat layer → SMAS → (premasseteric space) → parotidomasseteric fascia → parotid gland and masseter muscle → periosteum. It is tightly attached between the SMAS and masseteric fascia by masseteric cutaneous retaining ligaments. When ZCL, which originates from the inferior border of zygomatic arch to skin, is developed, it is likely to attached tightly, so when the filler is injected, it is likely not to elevate but spreads to the surrounding area, so it is recommended to apply subcision, release, and undermine before filler injection (Fig. 6-3-18).

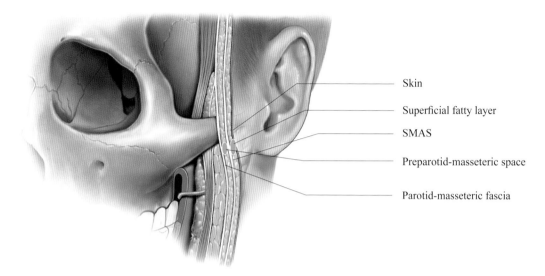

Skin

Superficial fatty layer

SMAS

Preparotid-masseteric space

Parotid-masseteric fascia

Fig. 6-3-18 Five anatomical layers of the lateral cheek area

The entry point would be the crossing point of the vertical line from the lateral orbital rim and virtual line from the oral commissure to tragus (Fig. 6-3-19). Insert the cannula, and release adhesions of the retaining ligaments; then, inject using the retrograde fanning technique. Inject as close to the zygomatic lower border as possible to avoid sunken creases.

Injection depth is the superficial fat layer; inject the filler at the deepest sunken part until the level of the zygomatic arch; then feather the surrounding area to avoid overcorrection. When there is severely depressed, release some ligaments between layers 3 and 5 using a cannula, and inject in the released space (maybe upper premasseteric space and some preparotid area). Most depressed areas are just below the zygomatic arch, so augment as close to the level of the zygomatic arch as possible and feather the lower part and gently massage to avoid bulging, lump, and irregularity. Additionally consider injecting the soft filler at the subdermal layer. Some might be concerned about parotid duct damage, but actually, parotidomasseteric fascia is a very tough structure and cannot even be denuded by a surgical knife, so using a cannula would be very safe, and even using a needle would be relatively safe unless injection is too deep. Parotid duct location is the medial 1/3 of the virtual line from the tragus and cheilion, and from that point, the horizontal line would be a pathway above the masseter muscle.

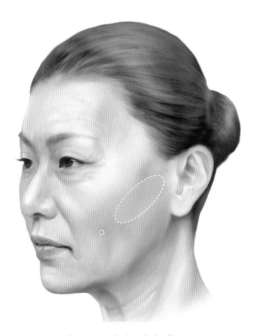

Fig. 6-3-19 Entry point for lateral cheek hollowness

Suggestive Readings

1. Mendelson BC, Jacobson SR. Surgical anatomy of the midcheek: facial layers, spaces, and the midcheek segments. Clinics in plastic surgery. 2008;35(3):395-404; discussion 393.
2. Mendelson BC, Muzaffar AR, Adams WP, Jr. Surgical anatomy of the midcheek and malar mounds. Plastic and reconstructive surgery. 2002;110(3):885-96; discussion 97-911.
3. Rohrich RJ, Pessa JE. The fat compartments of the face: anatomy and clinical implications for cosmetic surgery. Plastic and reconstructive surgery. 2007;119(7):2219-27; discussion 28-31.
4. Rohrich RJ, Pessa JE, Ristow B. The youthful cheek and the deep medial fat compartment. Plastic and reconstructive surgery. 2008;121(6):2107-12.

Lateral cheek augmentation at a glance

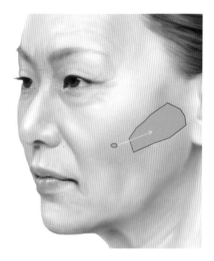

- Dr. Hyun-Jo Kim (Dermatologist)'s technique

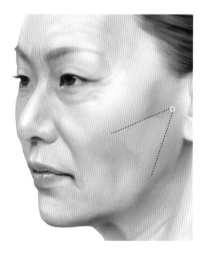

- Dr. Choon-Shik Youn (Dermatologist)'s technique

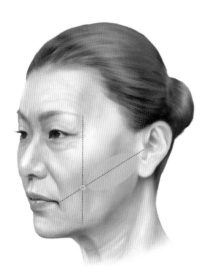 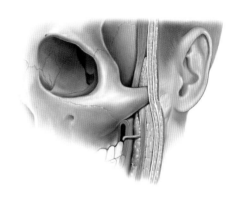

• **Dr. Gi-Woong Hong (Plastic Surgeon)'s technique**

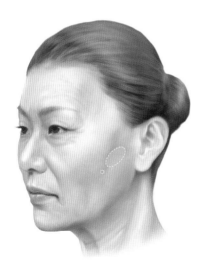 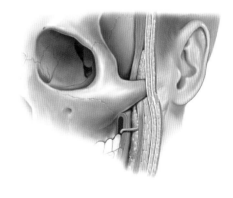

• **Dr. Eui-Sik Kim (Plastic Surgeon)'s technique**

	Dr. Kim HJ (Derma)	Dr. Youn (Derma)	Dr. Hong (PS)	Dr. Kim ES (PS)
Needle/cannula	23G cannula	23G cannula	21G or 23G cannula	23G cannula
Unilateral amount	1~2 mL	1~2 mL	Hard filler: 0.7~1 mL Soft filler: 0.2~0.3 mL	0.5~1 mL
Elasticity The Chaeum	No.2	No.4	Hard: No.3 Soft: No.1	Superficial: No.2 Deep: No.3
Anesthesia	EMLA cream	EMLA cream	EMLA cream and entry point local lidocaine Additional lidocaine when released	EMLA cream and entry point local lidocaine
Techniques	Fanning and linear threading technique	Fanning + linear threading technique	Deep: retrograde horizontal fanning and crossing technique, layer technique Superficial: linear threading and droplet technique	Release, undermine Retrograde fanning
Layer	Superficial fat (layer2)	Subcutaneous	Deep: premasseteric space between SMAS and parotid-masseteric fascia Superficial: subdermal layer	Layer 2 (subQ) Severe: + layer 4 (sub-SMAS space)

7-1 Nasolabial fold correction

Hyung-Ik Baik, M.D., Plastic Surgeon

7. 1. 1 Design

The nasolabial fold looks like a crease or a simple depression without crease. Moreover, it would look like a hill and valley stepladder and multiple wrinkles without crease or depression when smiling. All cases are called nasolabial folds but should be corrected differently.

There are multiple causes of nasolabial folds, and usually, they are combined.

When there is a congenitally depressed paranasal bone, the nasolabial fold would be shown before the aging process.

Lip elevators such as levator labii superioris alaeque nasi, levator labii superioris, zygomaticus major, and zygomaticus minor muscles originate from the bone and attach to the dermal layer of the nasolabial fold, so these are main causes of a deep crease or wrinkle.

Nasolabial fat, which is a superficial fat compartment, is located in the subcutaneous layer lateral to the nasolabial fold and would be one of the causes of deepening nasolabial fold when migrating downward during aging process. Deep medial cheek fat also decreases its volume during the aging process and might be a cause of prominent nasolabial fold (Fig. 7-1).

Deep fat compartment is the medial part of the deep medial cheek fat compartment, and there is Ristow's space between this fatty layer and the periosteum. Ristow's space is a safe and effective place to inject the filler.

The design should be different according to the shape and cause but generally performed as follows:

Draw a triangle as shown in Fig. 7-2; the bottom side should be at the alar base and the triangular apex to the oral commisure direction. The apex should be drawn until the depressed area when having a poker face. When smiling, the nasolabial wrinkle would be extended, so also draw an extended line.

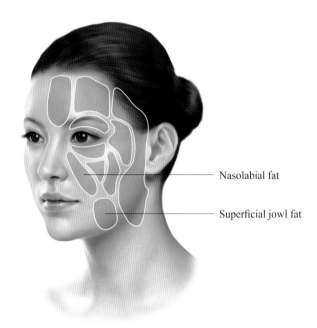

Nasolabial fat

Superficial jowl fat

Fig. 7-1 Superficial fat compartments of the face

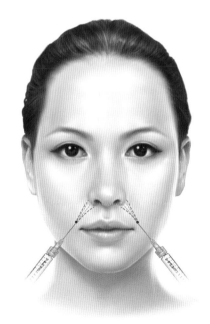

Fig. 7-2 Injection technique

A. Design triangle
B. Entry point
C. Insert a 23G 50 mm blunt cannula and inject the filler using the retrograde technique.

7. 1. 2 Anesthesia

EMLA cream application and local 1% lidocaine injection mixed with 1:200,000 epinephrine are performed. Lidocaine is injected at the entry point and Ristow's space or canine fossa minimally.

7. 1. 3 Techniques

7. 1. 3. 1 cannula

Using 23G 50 mm cannula by one entry point, inject the filler at Ristow's space (between deep medial cheek fat medial part and periosteum) or canine fossa.

The location of the entry point would not be on the design line but lateral to it, which is lateral to the triangular apex. That would be 1.5 cm lateral from the oral commissure and 1cm above.

Facial artery pathway is usually along the nasolabial fold, so intravascular filler injection might damage the large vessel or lead to severe complication. However, the needle is used just to puncture the skin, and the cannula is generally used so damage is avoided.

The relationship between the filler injection layer and facial artery running through the layer is more important.

There are few studies about facial artery depth, and there are controversies between Western and Oriental studies about facial artery depth, but there is no doubt that the deepest layer, which is the supraperiosteal layer, is the safest layer. Place the cannula tip to the desired site, and inject gently and a small amount retrogradely using the fanning technique.

Dynamic wrinkle is defined as a deeper nasolabial fold and/or extended fold when smiling or speaking. Injecting in the intradermal layer would solve these kinds of wrinkles.

Fig. 7-3 shows injection of Restylane Vital at the dermal layer using the fern-leaf or bridging technique.

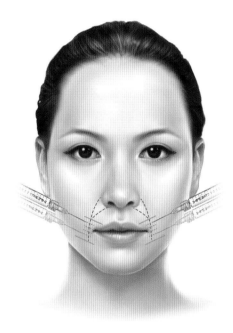

Fig. 7-3 Dermal injection

A. Improving dynamic wrinkle by soft filler
B. Inject in the superficial dermal layer using a 30G sharp needle
C. In the depressed area, inject at the medial side, and in the extended wrinkle, inject from the lateral side by the bridging technique.

When there is stepladder crease due to well-developed nasolabial fat, inject perpendicular to the wrinkle line using the fern-leaf technique, and the needle bevel should be in downward direction, and inject a very small amount of filler retrogradely.

When there are no stepladder wrinkles, a small amount of filler should be injected at the superficial dermis using the bridging technique.

After performing dermal injection, it is recommended to massage the area with a roller to prevent lump formation.

7. 1. 3. 2 Filler amount

The filler amount would be 1mL unilaterally when injected deeply at the supraperiosteal layer and approximately 0.2 mL unilaterally when injected at the dermal layer.

7. 1. 3. 3 Progress and photograph

There is almost no swelling, but check after 1 week for additional injection (Fig. 7-4, 7-5).

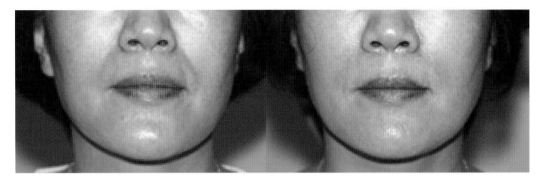

Fig. 7-4 Before and after

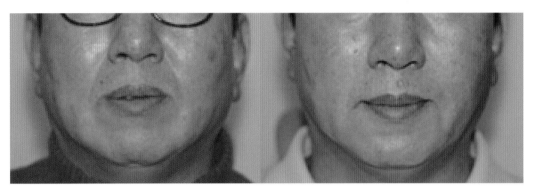

Fig. 7-5 Before and after

7. 1. 3. 4 Cautions

Common precautions in every filler injection are followed. The cannula or needle should not be antero-gradely injected, and the cannula or needle tip should be at the desired location, and retrograde injection should be performed. Moreover, do not inject a large amount of filler with high pressure, but inject a small amount gently multiple times.

7. 1. 3. 5 Complications and management

All complications of the filler would develop, and serious complications will be discussed.

Nodule or biofilm by hypersensitivity would develop, and treatment would be injection of hyaluronidase, steroids, or 5FU, and surgical management might also be needed.

These complications are thought to be caused by contamination, septic procedure, or inappropriate filler use.

The most serious problems are intraarterial embolism, skin necrosis along arterial territories, and blindness.

Skin necrosis does not develop immediately but 2~3 days after injection, and if there is erythema and pain in the injected or surrounding area, vascular compromise should be considered, and immediate hyaluronidase injection should be performed.

Suggestive Readings

1. Gierloff M, Stohring C, Buder T, Gassling V, Acil Y, Wiltfang J. Aging changes of the midfacial fat compartments: a computed tomographic study. Plastic and reconstructive surgery. 2012;129(1):263-73.
2. Rohrich RJ, Pessa JE, Ristow B. The youthful cheek and the deep medial fat compartment. Plastic and reconstructive surgery. 2008;121(6):2107-12.

Yong-Woo Lee, M.D., M.B.A., Plastic Surgeon

7. 2. 1 Design

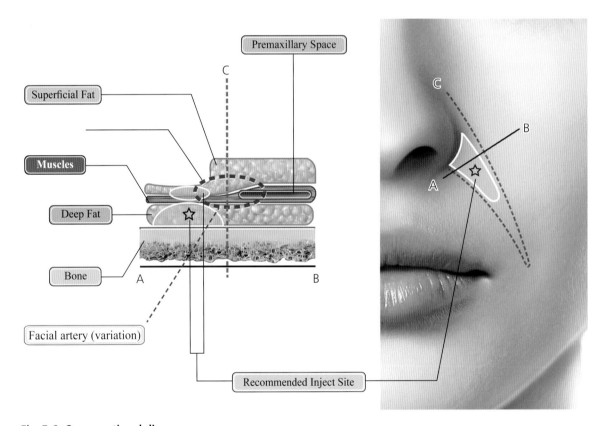

Fig. 7-6 Cross-sectional diagram

7. 2. 2 Anesthesia

Lidocaine subcutaneous injection is performed at the entry point located at the lateral end of the nasolabial fold.

7. 2. 3 Techniques

7. 2. 3. 1 Needle vs cannula

Inject using a 23G needle approaching 30~45° from the skin, inject gently as shown in Fig. 7-6 star marking just before touching the bone. When the patient feels electrical pain or skin bulging due to bleeding, insert the needle tip in a different pathway.

Lateral part of Fig. 7-6, line C, should be compressed hardly to avoid filler migration in the undesired area and vascular compromise.

7. 2. 3. 2 Filler amount

It is recommended that 70% of injection should be at the supraperiosteal layer; inject 0.2~0.3 mL and check Fig. 7-6 star marking whether it is properly injected.

It is recommended not to remove the needle tip but inject at the subcutaneous layer at the same entry point. Fig. 7-6 star marking is the same target region and would look unnatural when injection is performed too superficially.

7. 2. 3. 3 Cautions

DMCF is located at the supraperiosteal layer where the facial artery is seldom located. Thus, migration to undesired location should be considered only when the filler is injected deeply. When injecting at the subcutaneous layer, the facial artery would run in the same layer, so it is important to inject slowly with low pressure. It is important to compress the lateral side of the nasolabial fold because it might aggravate the fold when the filler migrates to the lateral side.

7. 2. 3. 4 Complications and management

The most serious complications are skin necrosis and visual complications. Especially, nasal alar necrosis could develop when lateral nasal artery obstruction develops. Moreover, the filler might run to the ophthalmic artery through the facial artery, and compression lateral to the line C might reduce this possibility.

Suggestive Readings

1. Brandt MG, Hassa A, Roth K, Wehrli B, Moore CC. Biomechanical properties of the facial retaining ligaments. Archives of facial plastic surgery. 2012;14(4):289-94.
2. Gierloff M, Stohring C, Buder T, Gassling V, Acil Y, Wiltfang J. Aging changes of the midfacial fat compartments: a computed tomographic study. Plastic and reconstructive surgery. 2012;129(1):263-73.
3. Lee JG, Yang HM, Choi YJ, Favero V, Kim YS, Hu KS, et al. Facial arterial depth and relationship with the facial musculature layer. Plastic and reconstructive surgery. 2015;135(2):437-44.
4. Mendelson B, Wong CH. Changes in the facial skeleton with aging: implications and clinical applications in facial rejuvenation. Aesthetic plastic surgery. 2012;36(4):753-60.
5. Wong CH, Mendelson B. Facial soft-tissue spaces and retaining ligaments of the midcheek: defining the premaxillary space. Plastic and reconstructive surgery. 2013;132(1):49-56.

Choon-Shik Youn, M.D., Dermatologist

7. 3. 1 Pathophysiology

1. Muscle fibers from the lip elevators attached to the dermis: there is a report that the maxillary ligament pulls the skin, but since the attachment site of the maxillary ligament does not coincide with the nasolabial fold, this report is controversial. Continuous movement of the lip elevator and attachment of the muscle fiber are the principal cause.

2. Superficial fat above the nasolabial fold drooping and deep fat, which is the DMCF, volume loss

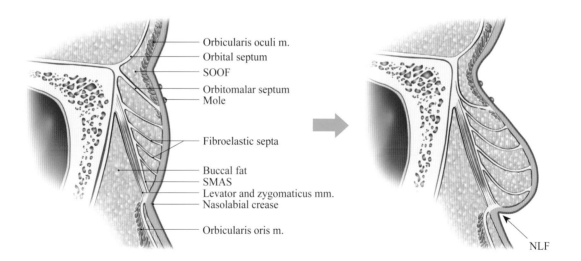

Orbicularis oculi m.
Orbital septum
SOOF
Orbitomalar septum
Mole

Fibroelastic septa

Buccal fat
SMAS
Levator and zygomaticus mm.
Nasolabial crease

Orbicularis oris m.

NLF

Fig. 7-7 Nasolabial fold: superficial fat sagging and DMCF volume loss

3. Differences in tissue density between the nasolabial fold medial and upper parts: the medial part is
dense and tight, while the upper part fatty tissues are loose (Fig. 7-8).

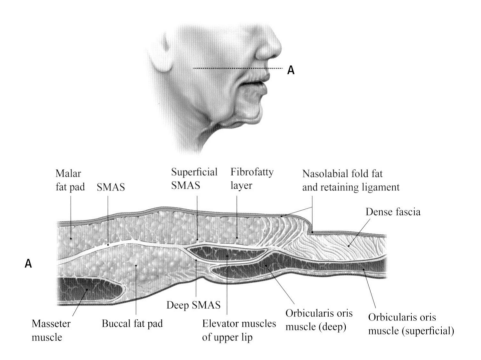

Fig. 7-8 **Nasolabial fold: differences in tissue density**

7. 3. 2 Design and surface anatomy

7. 3. 2. 1 Nasolabial fold classification by length: 1. Short, 2. extended, and 3. continuous

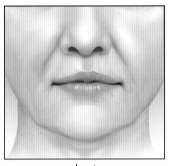 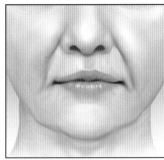 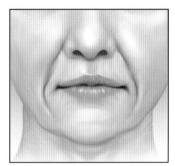

short   Extended   Continuous

Fig. 7-9 **Nasolabial fold: length**

7. 3. 2. 2 Nasolabial fold classification by shape: 1. Concave, 2. straight, and 3. convex

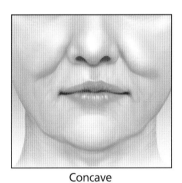 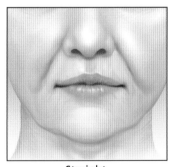 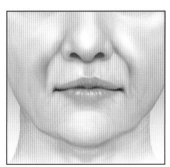

Concave   Straight   Convex

Fig. 7-10 **Nasolabial fold: shape**

7. 3. 2. 3 Design

Draw first the alar recess, which is the most augmented site, and then the line below.

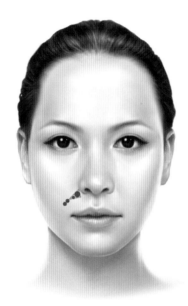

Fig. 7-11 Nasolabial fold: design

7. 3. 3 Anesthesia

7. 3. 3. 1 EMLA cream application: the author only uses EMLA cream.

7. 3. 3. 2 Lidocaine

Regional nerve block is not needed, and when a cannula is used, lidocaine is injected at the entry point.

7. 3. 4 Technique

7. 3. 4. 1 Needle or cannula

7. 3. 4. 1. 1 Needle: upper nasolabial fold (alar recess)

Inject at two layers, deep to the supraperiosteal or DMCF, and subcutaneous layer (layer2). Gierloff et al. described that DMCF crosses the nasolabial fold and evenly decreases volume during the aging process (Fig. 7-12). Thus, injection at the DMCF is very important. When injecting deeply, feel the bone and inject; when injecting superficially, inject at the subdermal layer to avoid the facial artery. The amount would depend on the depth, but usually 0.4 mL in deep wrinkle and 0.1 mL in superficial wrinkle at one point. When the wrinkle is shallow, just inject at the subdermal layer, and when it is deep, inject at two layers (Fig. 7-13). When injecting in a deep wrinkle, the ratio would be 1:1, and when a shallow line could be seen, intradermal injection is additionally performed.

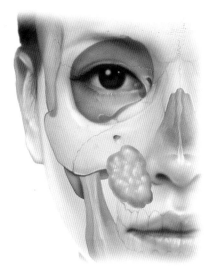

Fig. 7-12 Deep medial cheek fat:
medial fat of the deep medial cheek fat extends to the incisors, so injection at the DMCF would augment the nasolabial fold.

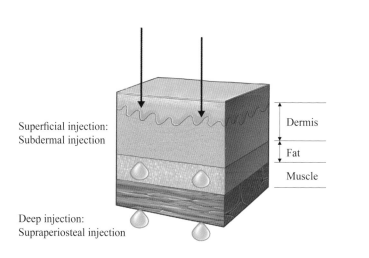

Superficial injection:
Subdermal injection

Dermis

Fat

Muscle

Deep injection:
Supraperiosteal injection

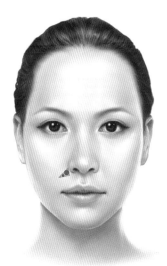

Fig. 7-13 Kisses technique: needle, superficial and deep injection

7. 3. 4. 1. 2 Needle: Lower nasolabial fold (lower than the alar recess)

Avoid the facial artery, and inject at the intradermal and subdermal layers using the vertical injection technique (Fig. 7-14)

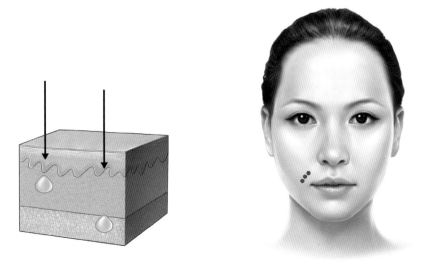

Fig. 7-14 Kisses technique: needle, intradermal and subdermal injection

7. 3. 4. 1. 3 Cannula

The target regions are two layers, subcutaneous and supraperiosteal layer. Make an entry point at the end of the nasolabial fold or the point that changes direction. When the entry point is punctured, feel the perforation in the dermal layer to avoid the facial artery.

Techniques are linear threading and fan technique at the subdermal layer of the alar recess and then linear threading techniques below the level of the alar recess. After subdermal injection, inject at the supraperiosteal layer at the DMCF (Fig. 7-15).

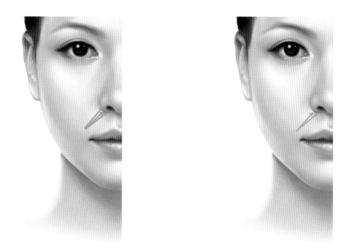

Fig. 7-15 Linear threading technique: cannula, superficial and deep injection

7. 3. 4. 2 Filler amount

The amount is usually 1~2 mL/side

7. 3. 4. 3 Progress and photograph

The deep nasolabial fold should be corrected by two-layer injection (subdermal and supraperiosteal layers).

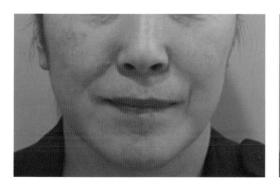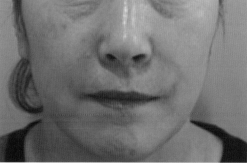

Fig. 7-16 Nasolabial fold: deep fold (two layers), before and 4 weeks after injection

Middle depth nasolabial fold is corrected by one-layer (subdermal) correction with a cannula.

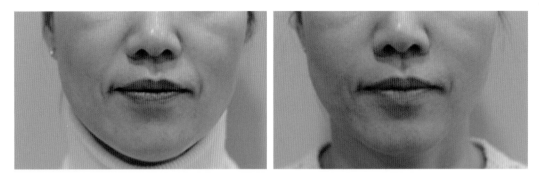

Fig. 7-17 **Nasolabial fold: middle depth fold (one layer), before and after**

Shallow nasolabial fold would be corrected at the subdermal layer using a needle.

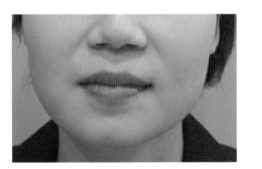 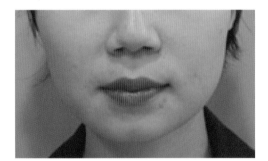

Fig. 7-18 **Nasolabial fold: shallow fold (one layer), before and after**

A case of multiple wrinkles and corrected nasolabial fold, perioral wrinkle, and Marionette line concomitantly

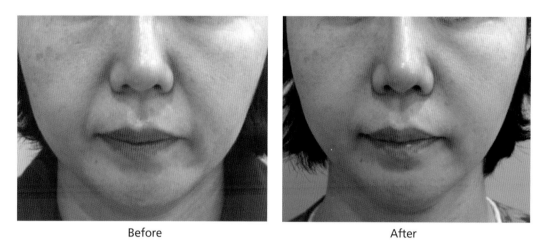

Before   After

Fig. 7-19 Nasolabial fold + perioral wrinkles + Marionette line: before and after

A case of not so deep nasolabial fold but with a crease. Subdermal or intradermal injection along the crease is recommended.

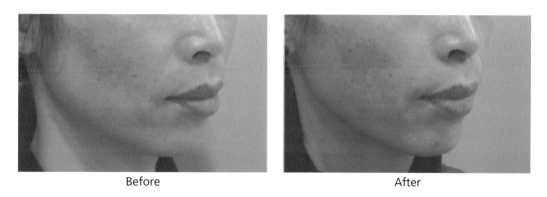

Before   After

Fig. 7-20 Nasolabial fold: only crease type, before and after

7. 3. 4. 4 Cautions

Nasolabial fold can be deep looking when injection is performed at the upper side of the crease or there is upward migration of filler by muscle action. Thus, care should be taken not to inject on the upper side.

There is some asymmetry of nasolabial fold before injection and the patient should be informed and different amount of injection should be considered (Fig. 7-21).

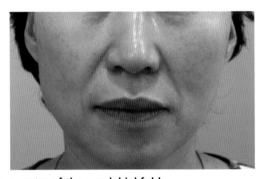

Fig. 7-21 Asymmetry of the nasolabial fold

When lip elevator power is high and the patient is smiling repeatedly, filler longevity could be reduced, so concomittant treatment is considered to inject botulinum toxin at the levator labii superioris alaeque nasi muscle.

Assess: Muscle movement

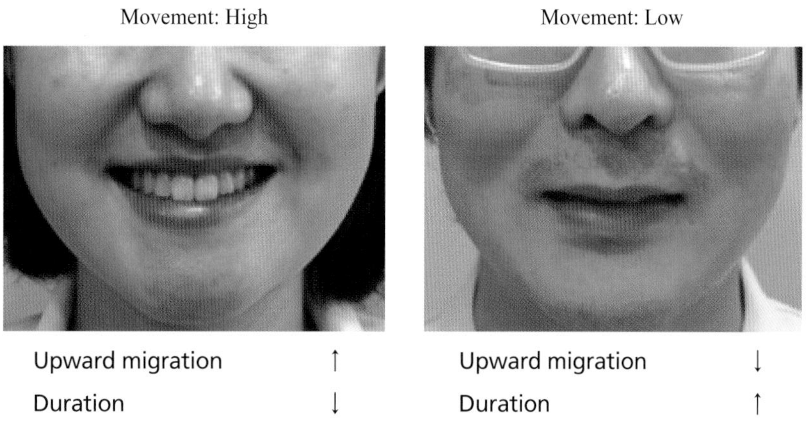

Movement: High | Movement: Low

| Upward migration | ↑ | Upward migration | ↓ |
| Duration | ↓ | Duration | ↑ |

Fig. 7-22 Lip elevator muscles

7. 3. 4. 5 Complications and management

The most severe complication is skin necrosis by facial artery damage. To avoid facial artery, the following should be performed:

1) depth

inject at the subdermal or supraperiosteal level to avoid facial artery.

2) gentle injection

To puncture the artery by a cannula, intravenous catheterization should be simulated. To perform IV, we stretch the tissue and puncture the needle abruptly, so when we inject in a vice versa method, which is gentle and slow injection, intravascular injection could be of low possibility.

7-4 Nasolabial fold

Yu-Ri Kim, M.D., Ph.D., Dermatologist

7. 4. 1 Design

Senile changes initially occur at the periocular and perioral region because many muscles are attached to the skin in this area, and this area is involved in several movements. Wrinkles are commonly observed at the nasolabial fold because of various movements and soft tissue volume changes. To correct the nasolabial fold, wrinkles, soft tissue volume, and excessive muscle movements should be assessed. Usually, dermal wrinkles and soft tissue are the problems.

Dermal wrinkles can be classified as dynamic and static wrinkles and by wrinkle pattern as wrinkle, fold, and crease (Fig. 7-23). In static wrinkles, the thickness of dermis decreased, so soft filler should be injected at the dermal layer.

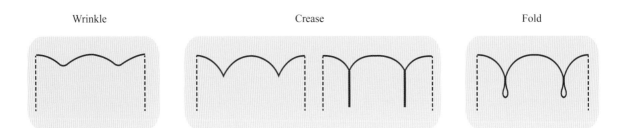

Wrinkle   Crease   Fold

Fig. 7-23 **Various wrinkle patterns**

Soft tissue changes in the aging process are usually caused by reduced volume of the deep fat compartment and bony recession. Sometimes, skin sagging could be observed because of increased nasolabial fat, which is a superficial fat compartment. Deep pyriform space (Ristow's space) extends from the depressor septi nasi muscle to the tear trough ligament vertically and from the deep medial cheek fat to the lobular connective tissue horizontally and is covered by the levator labii superioris muscle. This space is increased by the decreased volume of DMCF (deep medial cheek fat) and bony resorption in the aging process. Considering these facts, the nasolabial fold should be corrected by volumizing the deep fat compartment and deep pyriform space, and superficial fat should also be minimized by skin lifting using a thread.

7. 4. 2 Anesthesia

EMLA cream is adequate because many types of fillers contain lidocaine. It is suitable when making an entry point by an 18G needle puncture; however, lidocaine injection could be performed to reduce pain (Fig. 7-24).

7. 4. 3 Technique

7. 4. 3. 1 Needle

It is recommended not to use a needle at the subcutaneous layer because of many arterial variations, but in treating the dermal layer in a static wrinkle, injecting the soft filler by intradermal injection is recommended.

7. 4. 3. 2 Cannula

It is recommended to puncture at a site located laterally from the fold because the filler could seep out when the puncture is particularly near the entry point. The puncture depth should be 2~3 mm to avoid damaging adjacent vessels. A large-diameter cannula can be inserted through the entry point made by an 18G needle when puncturing vertically.

A small amount of the filler is needed to volumize the alar recess superficial fat layer, but lumps might develop. Moreover, tissues in the superficial fat layer are denser compared to those in the deep fat layer; therefore, the filler could migrate to the nasolabial fat compartment, and the nasolabial fold could be aggravated. To avoid this phenomenon, the cannula tip should be placed remarkably near the alar recess, and the cheek area should be compressed.

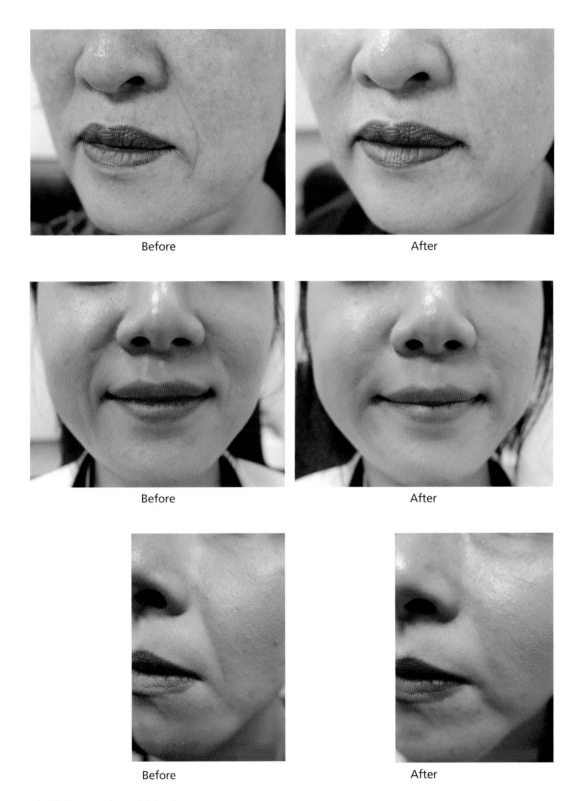

Before

After

Before

After

Before

After

Fig. 7-24 **Intradermal injection**

The cannula could be placed at the pyriform space after penetrating the alar side of the deep fat layer. Nasolabial folds can be corrected naturally when injecting at the deep pyriform space or deep fat layer, but a large amount of filler may be required.

7. 3. 4 Filler amount

There would be no pain or lumps when a large volume (1 mL/side) of the filler is injected at the deep pyriform space, but pain, lumps, or even migration might develop when a small volume (less than 0.5 mL/side) of the filler is injected at the subcutaneous layer.

Compression of the subcutaneous artery would occur even when a cannula is used. The angular artery is present at the septum between the deep pyriform space and deep medial cheek fat; therefore, it is relatively safe to inject at the deep fat layer.

7. 3. 5 Cautions

Patients are likely to expect correction of all wrinkles but should be informed of the extent of correction before treatment. It should be explained to the patient that concomitant correction of the anteromedial cheek is performed when this region is depressed. Moreover, when cheek sagging occurs, thread lifting should be considered.

Further, botulinum toxin injection should be considered when there are severe dynamic wrinkles.

Suggestive Readings

1. Surek CK, Vargo J, Lamb J. Deep Pyriform Space: Anatomical Clarifications and Clinical Implications. Plastic and reconstructive surgery. 2016;138(1):59-64.
2. Gierloff M, Stohring C, Buder T, Gassling V, Acil Y, Wiltfang J. Aging changes of the midfacial fat compartments: a computed tomographic study. Plastic and reconstructive surgery. 2012;129(1):263-73.

Nasolabial fold correction at a glance

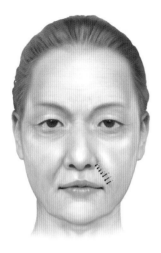

● **Dr. Hyun-Ik Baik (Plastic Surgeon)'s technique**

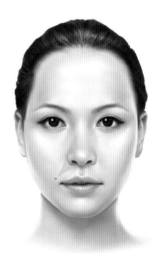

● **Dr. Yong-Woo Lee (Plastic Surgeon)'s technique**

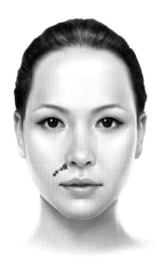

● **Dr. Choon-Shik Youn (Dermatologist)'s technique**

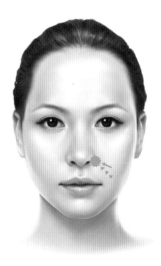

deep injection (arrow, orange),
intradermal injection (arrowhead, blue)

● **Dr. Yu-Ri Kim (Dermatologist)'s technique**

	Dr. Baik (PS)	Dr. Lee (PS)	Dr. Youn (Derma)	Dr. Kim (Derma)
Needle / cannula	Needle: 30G Cannula: 23G	Needle: 23G 1.25 in	Needle: 27G or 30G Cannula: 23G	Needle: 30G Cannula: 23G
Unilateral amount	Needle: 0.2 mL Cannula: 1 mL	0.5~1 mL	1~2 mL	1~2 mL
Elasticity The Chaeum	Needle: No.1 Cannula: No.3	No.3	Needle: No.3 Cannula: No.4	Needle: No.1 Cannula: No.3
Anesthesia	Local lidocaine injection	Local lidocaine injection	EMLA cream	EMLA cream / Local lidocaine injection
Techniques	1. Fern-leaf or bridging technique 2. Fanning technique	Bolus technique	Needle: vertical injection technique (Kisses technique) Cannula: fanning technique + linear threading technique	Intradermal layer: needle, blanching technique Deep fat layer: cannula, bolus technique
Layer	Superficial dermis Ristow's space (supraperiosteal layer)	Supraperiosteal layer Additionally, subdermal layer	Subcutaneous and supraperiosteal	Dermal layer Deep piriform space

CHAPTER **08**

Marionette's line, perioral wrinkle

8-1 Marionette line and perioral wrinkles

Yong-Woo Lee, M.D., M.B.A., Plastic Surgeon

MARIONETTE LINE

8. 1. 1 Design

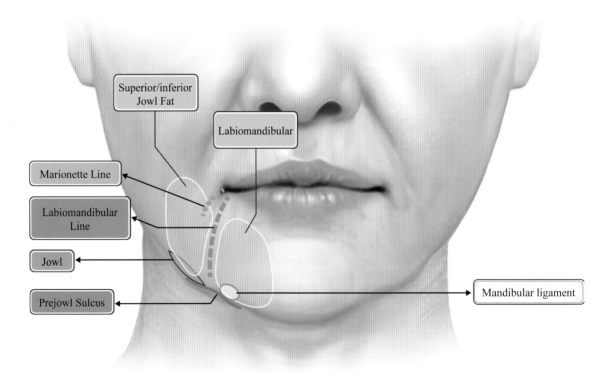

Fig. 8-1 **Anatomical borderline**

8. 1. 2 Anesthesia

Lidocaine injection is performed at the entry point that is located at the end of the marionette line at the lower border of the mandible.

8. 1. 3 Technique

8. 1. 3. 1 Needle versus cannula

Using a 23G needle, inject in an upward direction into the subcutaneous layer. It is also effective to inject diffusely in the triangular depressed area, which is at the medial side of the marionette line.

8. 1. 3. 2 Filler amount

The main cause is a marionette line medial area depression, and the lateral soft tissue of marionette line might show wrinkles. Thus, lateral part liposuction and/or lifting procedure would be the first choice to volumize the medial part. Injection at the subcutaneous layer is recommended, but when there is severe depression, injection into the layer deeper than the muscle might also be performed.

8. 1. 3. 3 Cautions

When filler injection is performed without correction of lateral soft tissue ptosis, there might be filler overdose, and an unexpected aesthetic result could be obtained. Therefore, correction using other procedures is recommended.

8. 1. 3. 4 Complications and management

Only a few complications develop. The facial artery runs deep, so there is a low possibility of damage. Collateral vessels are well developed, so there is a low possibility of skin necrosis. Visual complications rarely develop because the area is far from the eyes.

PERIORAL WRINKLES

8. 1. 4 Design

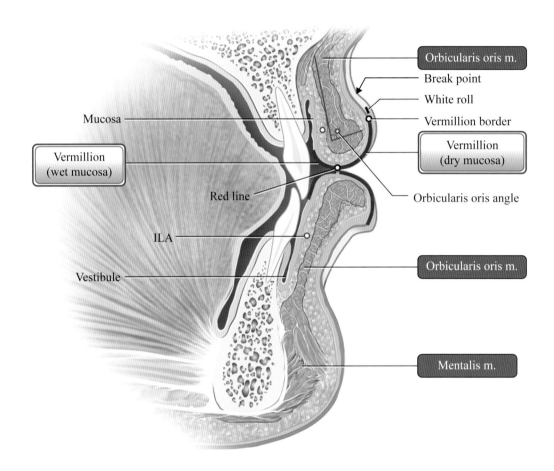

Orbicularis oris m.

Break point

White roll

Mucosa

Vermillion border

Vermillion
(dry mucosa)

Vermillion
(wet mucosa)

Red line

Orbicularis oris angle

ILA

Vestibule

Orbicularis oris m.

Mentalis m.

Fig. 8-2 **Sagittal view**

8. 1. 5 Anesthesia

When filler injection is performed outside the lip, inject lidocaine in the oral commissure entry points.

When filler inject is performed inside the mucosa of the lip, inject lidocaine in the mucosal area.

8. 1. 6 Technique

8. 1. 6. 1 Needle versus cannula

The 23G or 25G needle tip is placed at the central portion of the lip, and the filler is injected retrogradely.

8. 1. 6. 2 Filler amount

When injection is performed outside the lip, the vermilion border is augmented and immediate changes can be observed, and in this case, a relatively small amount of filler is needed. However, when injection is performed inside the mucosa, the filler should be placed just below the wet mucosa, making the lip flip over. In this case, double the amount of filler is needed.

8. 1. 6. 3 Cautions

Usually, injection is performed outside the vermilion border, but sometimes it is performed inside the mucosa. In Fig.8-2, the normal lip has a breakpoint, and the vermilion border reveals lip thickness from the frontal view. The breakpoint has a decreased angle and flattens during the aging process; thus, if flipping over of the lip is preferred, it is better to inject the filler in the mucosal side.

8. 1. 6. 4 Complications and management

Vascular complications are rare. The locations of the superior and inferior labial arteries should be determined. As shown in Fig. 8-2, both arteries run posterior to the orbicularis oris muscle, and the superior labial artery is located at the level of the filler injection height, which is near the lips, and the inferior labial artery tends to run lower and farther from both lips. Vascular compromise should be considered when injecting in the upper lips, especially in cases involving injections in the mucosa.

Suggestive Readings

1. Gierloff M, Stohring C, Buder T, Wiltfang J. The subcutaneous fat compartments in relation to aesthetically important facial folds and rhytides. Journal of plastic, reconstructive & aesthetic surgery : JPRAS. 2012;65(10):1292-7.

2. Mendelson B, Wong CH. Changes in the facial skeleton with aging: implications and clinical applications in facial rejuvenation. Aesthetic plastic surgery. 2012;36(4):753-60.

3. Penna V, Stark GB, Eisenhardt SU, Bannasch H, Iblher N. The aging lip: a comparative histological analysis of age-related changes in the upper lip complex. Plastic and reconstructive surgery. 2009;124(2):624-8.

4. Rohrich RJ, Pessa JE. The anatomy and clinical implications of perioral submuscular fat. Plastic and reconstructive surgery. 2009;124(1):266-71.

5. Tansatit T, Apinuntrum P, Phetudom T. A typical pattern of the labial arteries with implication for lip augmentation with injectable fillers. Aesthetic plastic surgery. 2014;38(6):1083-9.

Marionette line and perioral wrinkles

Hyung-Ik Baik, M.D., Plastic Surgeon

It is hard to choose one specific name for multiple wrinkles from the oral commissure to the chin. Perioral wrinkles have various shapes because of the direction, depth, and shapes of wrinkles are different due to multiple anatomical factors.

The author classified these wrinkles. Wrinkles that do not have hills and valleys are called lines, and those that have such features are called folds.

They are classified into two categories: First is the extended type of nasolabial fold, which is a nasolabial fold that does not connect to the oral commissure, but extends to the mentum area (Fig. 8-3).

Second is the labio-mandibular fold or line, which starts from the oral commissure to the mandibular area. The classical fold is the marionette line or fold, which runs from the oral commissure to the lateral direction (Fig. 8-4), and the pseudo-marionette fold is also a type of fold that is caused by ptosis of buccal fat or superficial jowl fat (Fig. 8-5).

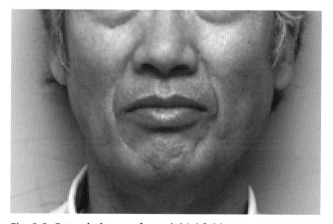

Fig. 8-3 **Extended type of nasolabial fold**

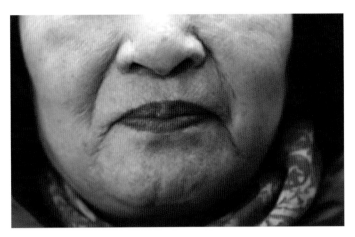

Fig. 8-4 **Typical marionette lines**

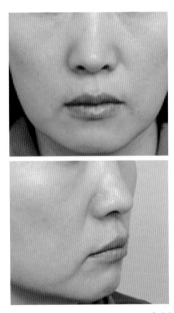

Fig. 8-5 **Pseudo-marionette fold**

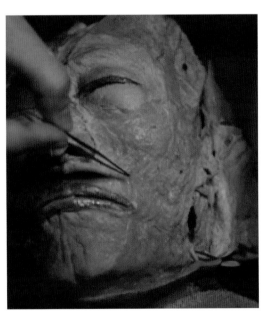

Fig. 8-6 **Location and shape of the depressor anguli oris**

The most associated anatomical structure is the depressor anguli oris (Fig. 8-6), and other factors are the zygomaticus major muscle bifid type, platysma muscle, risorius muscle, buccal fat pad, superficial jowl fat, and skin laxity.

8. 2. 1 Design

Various wrinkles develop, and several designs and techniques should be applied.

Here, we will describe the typical marionette line that is from the oral commissure to mandibular borderline.

In many cases, there are stepladder wrinkles caused by superficial jowl fat and show rectangular-shaped depression, as shown in Fig. 8-7, and the design for depressed prejowl sulcus is elliptical in shape.

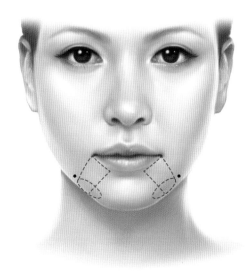

Fig. 8-7 Design for correction of marionette fold and depressed prejowl sulcus

8. 2. 2 Anesthesia

EMLA cream is applied, and 1% lidocaine with 1:200,000 epinephrine is injected at the entry point; the region filler is then injected.

8. 2. 3 Technique

8. 2. 3. 1 The appropriate filler for augmentation is injected using a 23G 50 mm cannula at one entry point. Inject the rectangular marionette area and prejowl sulcus using the fan technique (Fig. 8-8)**.**

The entry point should be slightly medial or lateral from the mandibular border, and lateral technique is more convenient.

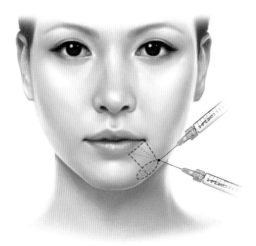

Fig. 8-8 Injection technique
(1) Entry point location
(2) 23G 50 mm blunt cannula filler injection
(3) fan technique, retrograde technique

It is recommended to inject the filler into the subcutaneous layer to avoid the inferior labial artery and mental nerve.

When there is a lack of subcutaneous fat, the filler can be injected under the most superficial mimetic muscle, which is the depressor anguli oris muscle, but care should be taken to avoid the structures described above.

To correct prejowl sulcus, both the supraperiosteal and subcutaneous layers are safe.

Locate the cannula tip, and gently inject a small amount of filler, unless there is a high possibility of bleeding and bruising.

The marionette line is also a dynamic wrinkle because it lengthens and deepens when smiling, so the appropriate filler (e.g., Restylane Vital) should be injected at the dermal layer and the filler amount could be reduced when deeply injected.

Inject at the superficial dermal layer with bevel down using the fern or bridging technique (Fig. 8-9).

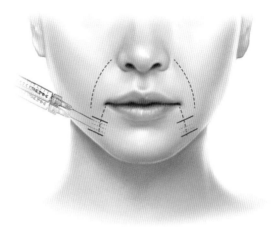

Fig. 8-9 Injection technique

(1) Soft filler
(2) inject at the superficial dermis using a 30G sharp needle
(3) when there is a fold, inject the filler medial from the marionette line
(4) when there is a line, inject the filler lateral from the marionette line using the bridging technique.

When there is stepladder fold caused by superficial jowl fat or deep buccal fat ptosis, inject perpendicular from the marionette line, placing the needle tip medial from the marionette line, and inject a small amount retrogradely.

When there is no stepladder fold and just dynamic wrinkles, inject the filler using the bridging technique.

After filler injection, flatten using a roller to prevent lumps.

If there is any lateral lip compartment depression, inject Restylane Vital at the medial side of the marionette line subdermal layer using a 30G needle.

At the perioral region, there would be various types of smile lines in the zygomaticus major, risorius, platysma, and depressor anguli oris muscles. These wrinkles develop with facial expression or during talking but could be in a static state when the wrinkle develops for a long time.

Vertical dermal injection by soft filler using a 30G needle could be performed. When the skin is thin with small amount of subcutaneous fat, inject the soft filler using a 27G cannula perpendicular to the wrinkles.

8. 2. 3. 2 Total amount to correct the marionette line and prejowl sulcus should not exceed 1 mL/side.

The amount to be injected in the dermal layer should be approximately 0.3 mL/side.

8. 2. 3. 3 Progress and photograph

Additional dermal injection could be performed after 1 week.

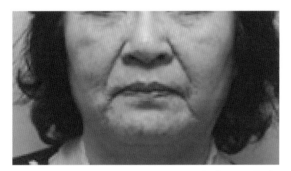 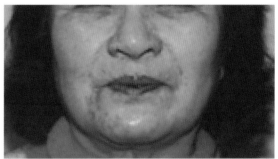

Fig. 8-10 Marionette line correction: before and after

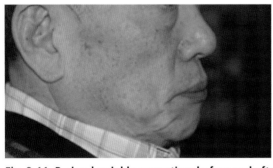 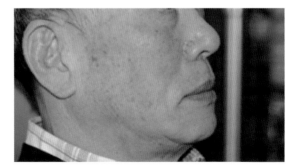

Fig. 8-11 Perioral wrinkle correction: before and after

8. 2. 3. 4 Cautions

The periorbital area is a common site for bruising; therefore, it is recommended to use a cannula unless injecting in the dermal layer. Although a cannula is used, the procedure should be performed carefully. Lumps might develop when a large amount is used in the dermal injection; thus, injection of a very small amount is recommended with repetition of the procedure after a week.

8. 2. 3. 5 Complications

Damage to the inferior labial artery or mental nerve might occur but very rarely.

Precise injection is required owing to occasional bruising.

Suggestive Readings

1. Pessa JE, Zadoo VP, Garza PA, Adrian EK, Jr., Dewitt AI, Garza JR. Double or bifid zygomaticus major muscle: anatomy, incidence, and clinical correlation. Clinical anatomy (New York, NY). 1998;11(5):310-3.

8-3 Marionette line and perioral wrinkles

Choon-Shik Youn, M.D., Dermatologist

8. 3. 1 Pathophysiology of the marionette line

1. Mandibular retaining ligament: this is a true ligament from the mandible to the skin, and upper structures do not migrate downward but develop folds.

2. Descent migration of buccal fat: the platysma and masseteric cutaneous ligament, which are supporting the fat in the buccal space, are loosened, and buccal fat migrates downward and augments the upper portion of the marionette line, resulting in a more depressed look (Fig. 8-12).

3. Descent migration of superficial fat: similar to nasolabial fat descent, jowl fat also migrates downward during the aging process.

4. Bone absorption: the mandibular retaining ligament attaches to a portion of the mandibular bone, which absorbs more than the other portions, so the prejowl sulcus and the marionette line deepen.

5. The volume of the labio-mandibular fat, which is located at the medial side of the marionette line, decreases.

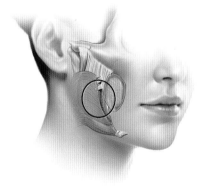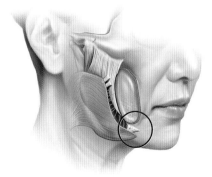

Fig. 8-12 **Jowl, marionette line, and prejowl sulcus**

* Perioral wrinkles are not related to the nasolabial fold but develop by continuous movement of the lip elevator and risorius muscles.

8. 3. 2 Surface anatomy

8. 3. 2. 1 Perioral wrinkles are fine wrinkles located lateral to nasolabial folds.

8. 3. 2. 2 The marionette line is a wrinkle from the lip commissure to the prejowl sulcus (Fig. 8-13).

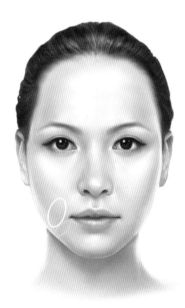

Fig. 8-13 Surface Anatomy: Perioral wrinkles(white) Marionette line(yellow)

8. 3. 3 Design

Perioral wrinkles and the marionette line are more prominently seen when smiling, so the design is made at the smiling position.

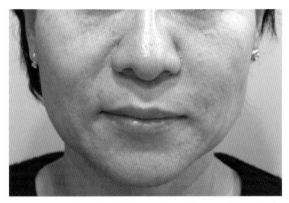 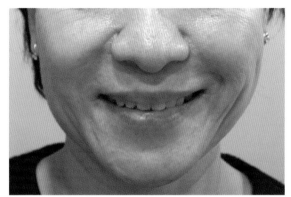

Fig. 8-14 **Perioral wrinkles and marionette line: design**

8. 3. 4 Anesthesia

The author performs EMLA cream application.

8. 3. 5 Technique

8. 3. 5. 1 Needle or cannula

The author almost always uses a needle to correct perioral wrinkles and the marionette line using the vertical injection technique.

8. 3. 5. 2 Depth

To avoid the facial artery and prevent dermal wrinkles, inject the filler at the subdermal layer and deep dermis.

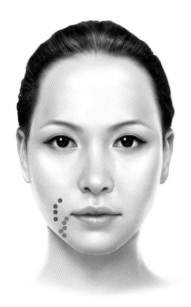
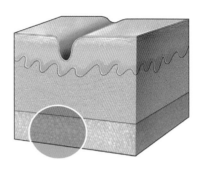

Fig. 8-15 **Perioral wrinkle and marionette line: kisses technique**

8. 3. 6 Filler amount

The average filler amount is 1~2 mL unilaterally.

8. 3. 7 Progress and photograph

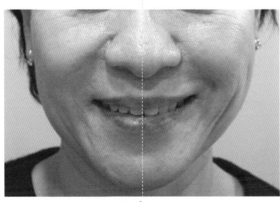
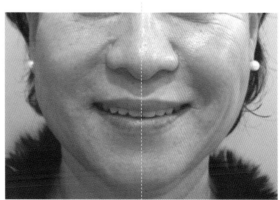

Before   5 weeks after

Fig. 8-16 **Perioral wrinkles and marionette line: before and after five weeks**
Rt : Elravie light (20 mg/mL) : 1.4 mL
Lt : Belotero balance (22.5 mg/mL) : 1.4 mL

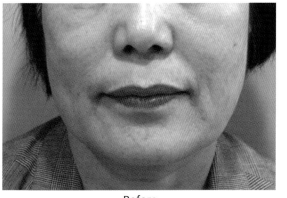 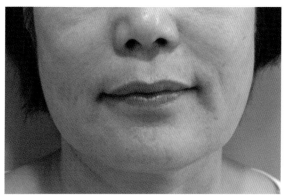

| Before | After |

Fig. 8-17 Perioral wrinkles and marionette line: before and after

Belotero balance: 1 mL/side, Belotero intense: 0.3 mL/side

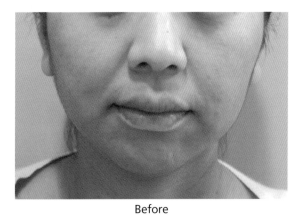 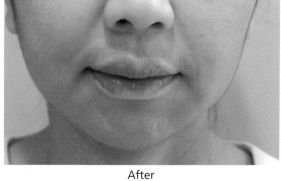

| Before | After |

Fig. 8-18 Marionette line: before and after

Belotero balance: 2.2 mL/side, Belotero intense: 0.7 mL/side

8. 3. 8 Cautions

Bruising often develops in the region, so the filler should be injected precisely into the intradermal or subdermal layer.

8. 3. 9 Complications and management

The winding portion of the facial artery, which is not covered by muscles and runs subcutaneously, is located in this area, so the filler should be injected only at the deep dermis or subdermal layer.

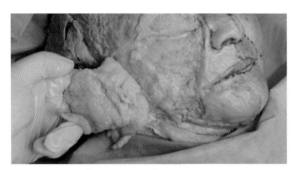 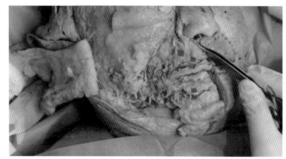

Fig. 8-19 Facial artery: winding portion

8-4 Marionette line and perioral wrinkles

Hyun-Jo Kim, M.D., M.S., Dermatologist

8. 4. 1 Design

The marionette line is known to be caused by depressor anguli oris muscle (Fig. 8-20) insertion, aging-related atrophy of the dermis, fat volume change, and migration of fatty tissue.

In contrast, perioral wrinkles are thought to be caused by orbicularis oris muscle insertion and aging-related atrophy of the dermis.

Design at the medial part of marionette line, which is the region with greatest volume loss (Fig. 8-21).

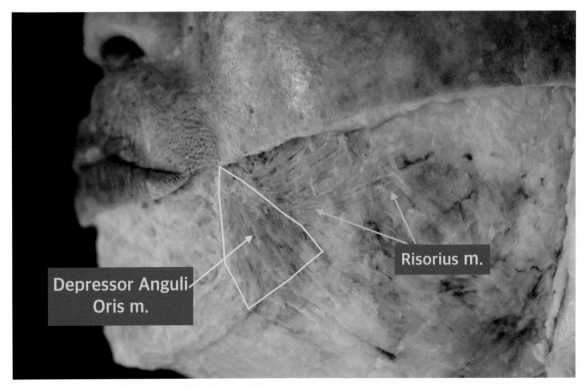

Fig. 8-20 **Marionette line surrounding the muscles**

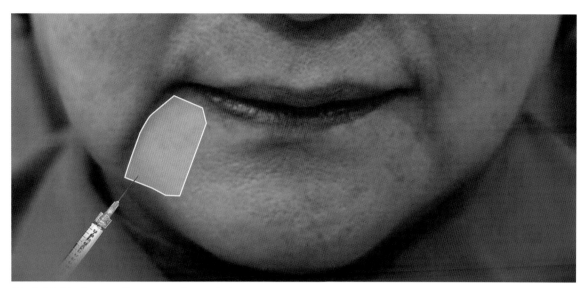

Fig. 8-21 Marionette line correction technique

Perioral wrinkles are static and dynamic; thus, two situations should be considered: when the area is depressed by volume loss, filler should be injected, and when there is excessive muscle action, botulinum toxin should be injected.

8. 4. 2 Anesthesia

EMLA cream is enough, and regional nerve block such as infraorbital or mental nerve block is helpful.

8. 4. 3 Technique

8. 4. 3. 1 Needle versus blunt-tip microcannula

The author prefers to use the needle. To correct the marionette line, both subcutaneous fat and periosteum layers can be injected, but in the case of injection into the periosteum, the amount to be injected should be 20~30% more.

Filler injection to correct perioral wrinkles is performed at the subcutaneous layer along the vermilion border, and 0.5~1 U botulinum toxin injection is performed along the vermilion border at points that are 1cm apart.

8. 4. 3. 2 Filler amount

To correct the marionette line, 0.5~1 mL of filler is needed unilaterally, and to correct perioral wrinkles, unlike lip augmentation, a small amount is needed. Overcorrection could lead to irregularity.

Perioral wrinkles usually develop in the upper lip, so when injecting along the vermilion border, 0.3~0.5 mL of filler is needed.

8. 4. 3. 3 Progress and photograph

Marionette line correction by injection at subcutaneous fat layer (Fig. 8-22).

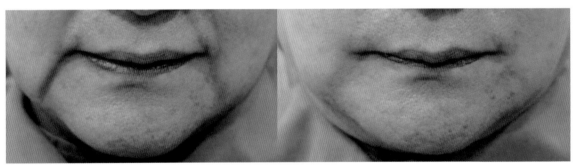

Fig. 8-22 Marionette line correction: before and after

8. 4. 3. 4 Cautions

The inferior labial artery is located between the depressor anguli oris muscle and depressor labii inferioris muscle. To avoid this vessel, injection should be performed into either the subcutaneous or periosteum layer (Fig. 8-23).

When the filler is injected in the upper lip, the superior labial artery runs posterior to the orbicularis oris muscle, and to avoid this vessel, the filler should be injected in the muscle layer or anterior to the muscle (Fig. 8-24). When the injection performed posterior to the muscle, it might damage the superior labial artery (Fig. 8-25).

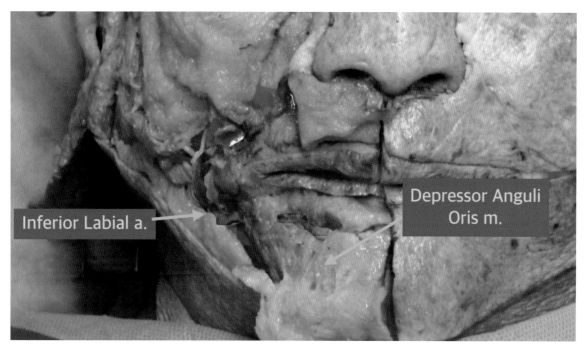

Fig. 8-23 **Marionette line: vessel in danger**

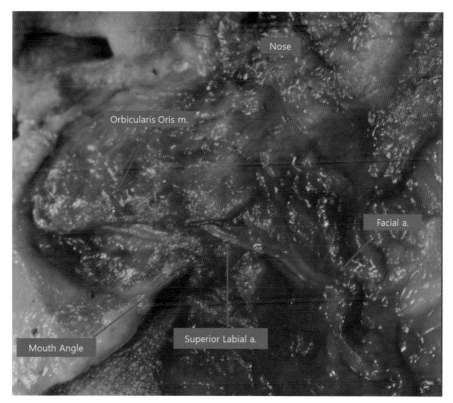

Fig. 8-24 **Superior labial artery location**

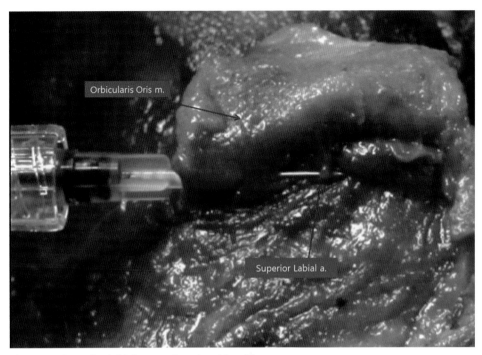

Fig. 8-25 Superior labial artery location (depth)

Suggestive Readings

1. LaTrenta GS. Atlas of Aesthetic Face & Neck Surgery: Saunders; 2004.
2. Lee SH, Lee M, Kim HJ. Anatomy-based image processing analysis of the running pattern of the perioral artery for minimally invasive surgery. The British journal of oral & maxillofacial surgery. 2014;52(8):688-92.
3. Yang HM, Lee JG, Hu KS, Gil YC, Choi YJ, Lee HK, et al. New anatomical insights on the course and branching patterns of the facial artery: clinical implications of injectable treatments to the nasolabial fold and nasojugal groove. Plastic and reconstructive surgery. 2014;133(5):1077-82.

Marionette line correction at a glance

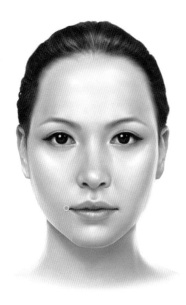

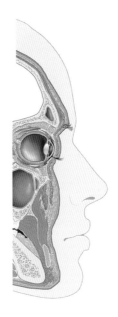

• **Dr. Yong-Woo Lee (Plastic Surgeon)'s technique**

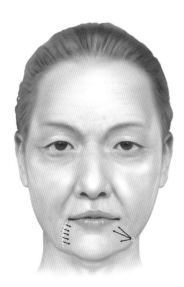

• **Dr. Hyung-Ik Baik (Plastic Surgeon)'s technique**

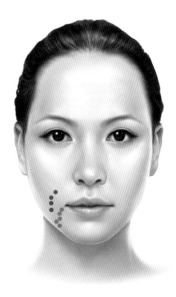

• **Dr. Choon-Shik Youn (Dermatologist)'s technique**

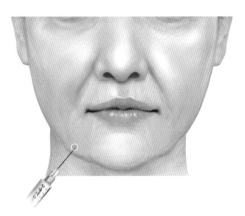

• **Dr. Hyun-Jo Kim (Dermatologist)'s technique**

Marionette line

	Dr. Lee (PS)	Dr. Baik (PS)	Dr. Youn (Derma)	Dr. Kim (Derma)
Needle/cannula	Cannula 23G	Cannula 23G	Cannula 21G or 23G	Cannula 23G
Unilateral amount	Less than 0.5 mL	Needle: 0.2 mL Cannula: 1 mL	1~1.5 mL	0.5~1.5 mL
Elasticity The Chaeum	No. 2	Needle: No. 1 Cannula: No. 3	No. 1 or 2	No. 2 or 3
Anesthesia	Local lidocaine injection	Local lidocaine injection	EMLA cream application	EMLA cream application
Techniques	Bolus technique	1. Fern or bridging technique 2. Fan technique	Vertical injection technique (kisses technique)	Linear threading and fan technique
Layer	Deep subcutaneous layer	1. Superficial dermis 2. Supraperiosteal layer	Deep dermis or subdermal layer	Periosteum or subcutaneous layer

Perioral wrinkles

	Dr. Lee (PS)	Dr. Baik (PS)	Dr. Youn (Derma)	Dr. Kim (Derma)
Needle/cannula		Needle 30G		Needle 33G
Unilateral amount		0.5 mL		0.5~0.8 mL
Elasticity The Chaeum	Same as that in the marionette line	No. 1	Same as that in the marionette line	No. 1 or 2
Anesthesia		EMLA cream application		EMLA cream application
Techniques		Fern or bridging technique		Linear threading and bolus(point) technique
Layer		Superficial dermis		Subcutaneous layer

Nose

Ee-Seok Lim, M.D., Ph.D., Dermatologist

9. 1. 1 Design

It is greatly important to check for nasal bone protrusion by inspection and palpation and decide whether the whole nose should be augmented or only the nasal root or tip.

9. 1. 2 Anesthesia

EMLA cream is used because the filler contains lidocaine. When a cannula is used, local lidocaine injection at the entry point is possible.

9. 1. 3 Technique

9. 1. 3. 1 Cannula versus needle

Use a 23G 5 cm cannula, which is relatively hard. A cannula that is too thin or too long can be difficult to handle.

In case of filler injection on just the nasal root or alar area, the author uses 0.3 mL insulin syringe. When using an insulin syringe to augment the nasal root area, the needle tip can be placed at the supraperiosteal layer, and a small amount of filler can be injected, so a safe and delicate procedure could be performed.

9. 1. 3. 2 Filler amount and property

A hyaluronic acid filler and relative hard biphasic filler are used, but an appropriate filler can be chosen for convenience.

For whole nasal area augmentation, 0.3~0.7 mL is usually used. When injection is performed at the root only, 0.2~0.4 mL is used, and at the nasal tip, 0.1~0.2 mL is used, but the amount depends on the patient's status.

9. 1. 3. 3 Technique

9. 1. 3. 3. 1 All dorsum

Inject lidocaine at the entry point and the filler in the supine position. Using a 23G 5 cm cannula, make an entry point at the infralobule, and insert the cannula tip in the nasal root. Inject the filler from sellion to nasal tip using a linear retrograde technique. The filler should be injected at the supraperiosteal layer, and check the location of the filler using the hand that is not holding the syringe. When the cannula tip crosses the point between the cartilage and bone, pull the cannula tip downward toward the supraperiosteal layer. This procedure is performed to avoid vascular compromise, which leads to skin necrosis and blindness, and when there is a bony hump, it is better to inject on the upper and lower portions separately.

9. 1. 3. 3. 2 Nasal root

The author uses a 0.3 mL insulin syringe. Inject perpendicular to the skin, and after touching the bone, inject the filler at the supraperiosteal layer. The root skin is thin and not tightly attached to the SMAS, so there is a relatively low possibility of compression skin necrosis. Aspirate to check for blood and then inject.

9. 1. 3. 3. 3 Nasal tip

Inject using a 23G 5 cm cannula between the lower lateral cartilage and supraperichondrial layer. The nasal tip area is composed of thick skin and tightly connected to the SMAS, so if there is excessive amount of filler, compression skin necrosis might develop. Never inject a large volume.

9. 1. 3. 4 Cautions

Nose vasculatures should be determined. It is composed of skin, superficial fatty layer, fibromuscular layer, deep fat layer and periosteum, and perichondrium. Among these, the fibromuscular layer is connected to the surrounding nasal muscles and located between the superficial and deep fat. The main vessels run at the fibromuscular layers, so to prevent vascular compromise, injection should be performed at the deeper fat layer.

9. 1. 3. 5 Complications and management

Blindness is recently a frequently occurring complication and is caused by injection of the filler at the dorsal nasal artery, regurgitating to the intraocular vessels. The causes might be physician malpractice, patient's abnormal vasculature, and superficial injection for more effective results. The author always injects at the supraperiosteal layer because safety is the most important and pinches the dorsum with two fingers of the contralateral hand. Always aspirate before injection. Do not use a large amount of filler at nasal tip. Check for pain and any skin color change.

Suggestive Readings

1.　Kim H-J, Seo KK, Lee H-K, Kim J. Clinical Anatomy of the Face for Filler and Botulinum Toxin Injection: Springer; 2016.
2.　Ozturk CN, Larson JD, Ozturk C, Zins JE. The SMAS and fat compartments of the nose: an anatomical study. Aesthetic plastic surgery. 2013;37(1):11-5.
3.　Tansatit T, Moon HJ, Rungsawang C, Jitaree B, Uruwan S, Apinuntrum P, et al. Safe Planes for Injection Rhinoplasty: A Histological Analysis of Midline Longitudinal Sections of the Asian Nose. Aesthetic plastic surgery. 2016;40(2):236-44.

Yong-Woo Lee, M.D., M.B.A., Plastic Surgeon

9. 2. 1 Design

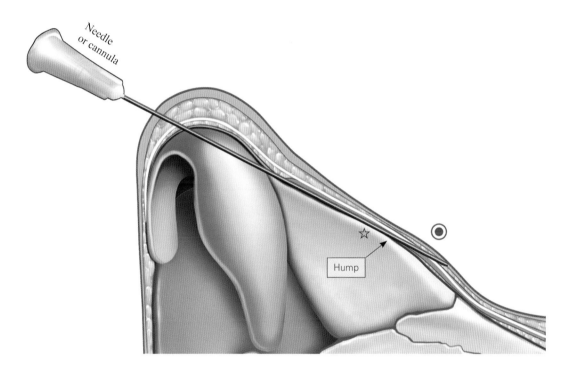

Fig. 9-1 Sagittal view of the nose

9. 2. 2 Anesthesia

Lidocaine injection is performed at the entry point.

9. 2. 3 Technique

9. 2. 3. 1 Needle versus cannula

A 21~23G 3.1~3.8 cm needle or 23G cannula 4~5 cm is used. It should just fit the length of the nose and not have a small diameter. The reasons for this are as follows: first, when we use a small-diameter needle, it is difficult to control the needle tip, and it could not be placed on the desired layer. When the syringe should be pulled upward, a small needle is likely to bend. The same phenomenon would occur in a very long needle (Fig. 9-1). Moreover, when we use a small-diameter needle, it is likely to be inserted into the vessel and could cause arterial regurgitation.

9. 2. 3. 2 Filler amount

For the dorsum of the nose, 0.4~0.7 mL of filler is used, and for the nasal tip, 0.1~0.3 mL. Always try to inject at the supraperichondial layer, and when additional injection is needed, inject a very small amount at the subdermal layer.

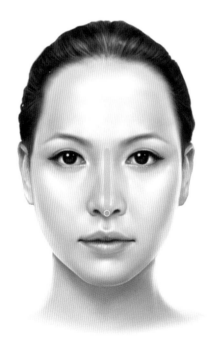

Fig. 9-2 Design and entry point

9. 2. 3. 3 Cautions

It is quite difficult to inject when there is a nose hump. The first method would be to make two entry points: below the hump area from the infralobule entry point and the nasal root area with another entry point to inject downward above the hump. The second method is to make just one entry point, but in this case, a long and thin cannula should not be used. Moreover, when passing through the hump area, the needle tip should be placed at the supraperiosteal layer. Another concern is that, after filler injection of the nose, the filler is likely to spread. Spreading is easy using molding procedure, but the reverse is very difficult.

9. 2. 3. 4 Complications

The nose is one of the most common areas of severe complication such as skin necrosis or visual disturbance. Skin necrosis often develops by increasing pressure between tight tissues and hard tissue such as the bone or cartilage. The alar area is supplied by the lateral nasal artery, and when this vessel is damaged, skin necrosis is likely to develop. The most severe complications are visual disturbances. This is because the dorsal nasal artery is a branch of the internal carotid artery and adjacent to the ophthalmic artery, and the distance is very short. It is relatively safe to compress the root area by the non-injecting hand. Moreover, carefully observe for skin color changes when injecting, and specially inject at the nasal tip area.

Suggestive Readings

1. Ha RY, Nojima K, Adams WP, Jr., Brown SA. Analysis of facial skin thickness: defining the relative thickness index. Plastic and reconstructive surgery. 2005;115(6):1769-73.
2. Kim P, Ahn JT. Structured nonsurgical Asian rhinoplasty. Aesthetic plastic surgery. 2012;36(3):698-703.
3. Kurkjian TJ, Ahmad J, Rohrich RJ. Soft-tissue fillers in rhinoplasty. Plastic and reconstructive surgery. 2014;133(2):121e-6e.
4. Ozturk CN, Larson JD, Ozturk C, Zins JE. The SMAS and fat compartments of the nose: an anatomical study. Aesthetic plastic surgery. 2013;37(1):11-5.
5. Saban Y, Andretto Amodeo C, Bouaziz D, Polselli R. Nasal arterial vasculature: medical and surgical applications. Archives of facial plastic surgery. 2012;14(6):429-36.

Nasal augmentation at a glance

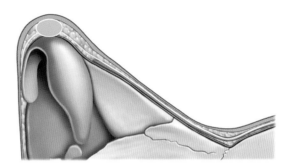

• Dr. Ee-Seok Lim (Dermatologist)'s technique

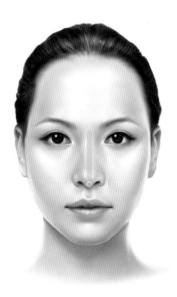

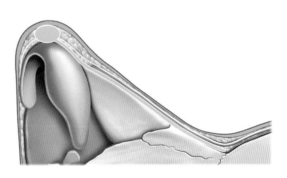

• Dr. Yong-Woo Lee (Plastic Surgeon)'s technique

	Dr. Lim (Derma)	Dr. Lee (PS)
Needle/cannula	Cannula 23G, 5 cm	Cannula 23G, 5 cm
Unilateral amount	0.3~0.5 mL	0.5~0.8 mL
Elasticity The Chaeum	No. 4	No. 3
Anesthesia	EMLA cream application	Local lidocaine injection
Techniques	Linear retrograde technique	Bolus
Layer	Supraperiosteal layer	Supraperiosteal layer, A Additional minimal filler above the SMAS, B

Lips

10-1 Lips

Jeong-Jun Park, M.D., Ph.D., Plastic Surgeon

10. 1. 1 Considerations before injection

Beautiful lips should have prominent borderline, be pinkish color and shiny, and have 2 mm protrusion in the upper lip than the lower lip. Laterally, the nasolabial angle should be obtuse. However, in the aging process, lip borders tend to obscure, wrinkles increase, and contour line tends to straighten.

The upper and lower lip volume ratio should be 1:1.5. When injection is performed, place the patient in a half-sitting position, and inject in the lower lip first.

It is recommended to inject less than 0.5~1 mL at one time.

10. 1. 2 Anatomical considerations

The layers of the lip include the skin, subcutaneous fat layer, orbicularis oris muscle layer, submuscular layer, and mucosal layer (Fig. 10-1).

In the frontal view, the lip can be divided into the skin and vermilion parts. The borderline between them is called white line. The vermilion part is again divided into dry and wet mucosa, and the junction is called dry-wet mucosal junction. The dermal layer would be the target for filler injection when the borderline is not prominent or smoker's line does not improve in the aging process. When a soft filler is injected along the white line, the borderline becomes prominent and the smoker's line improves. However, the ascending philtral artery runs at the philtral column, so care should be taken not to inject the filler deeply. The subcutaneous layer is a relatively safe layer because there are no delicate structures. The orbicularis oris muscle (OOM) is located under the subcutaneous fat layer. The OOM extends and attaches to the mucosa at the dry-wet mucosal junction. In the sagittal view, young people tend to have J-shaped lip eversion. During the aging process, it flattens to an I shape. Subcutaneous fat is located between the OOM and mucosa, and the superior labial artery, inferior labial artery, mental nerve, and labial glands are found in this layer. An important consideration about filler injection is that the labial artery runs at the subcutaneous fat that is attached to the wet mucosa. Thus, care should be taken when injecting through the mucosa.

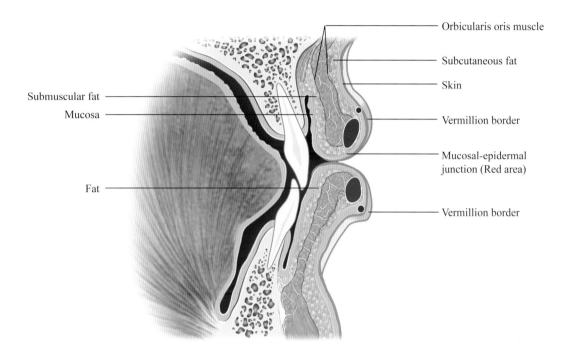

Submuscular fat

Mucosa

Fat

Orbicularis oris muscle

Subcutaneous fat

Skin

Vermillion border

Mucosal-epidermal junction (Red area)

Vermillion border

Fig. 10-1 Sagittal section of the lip

10. 1. 3 Technique

10. 1. 3. 1 Design: adjacent to the oral commissure

10. 1. 3. 2 Anesthesia

The lip are an extremely sensitive area, so EMLA cream application or regional nerve block is needed. Regional nerve block would be infraorbital or mental nerve block.

10. 1. 3. 3 Technique

The lips are soft, flexible, and sensitive. Thus, soft filler should be used instead of hard filler for tissue integrity. Hard filler is good for volumization but might cause an irregular shape or foreign body sensation.

To enhance the lip borderline, inject at the dermal or subdermal layer along the white line. A cannula is more difficult to use when injecting at the dermal layer (Fig. 10-2).

To change the shape or volumize the lip, it is recommended to use a cannula. The entry point would be considered to avoid the superior and inferior labial artery (Fig. 10-2). Thus, the entry point would be the oral commissure, and a cannula is used. It is known that 85% of facial artery branches are inside the virtual square of 1.5 cm lateral to and 1.5 cm above the oral commissure. Therefore, injecting under the OOM is quite dangerous. Use an 18G needle to make an entry point, and insert the cannula below the subcutaneous layer of the dry mucosa to midline. Inject the filler slowly by linear threading and retrograde fanning technique and be careful not to create fullness at the mouth corner. When the upper lip corner covers the lower lip, filler can be injected for lower lip corner augmentation to move the mouth corner upward. The lips should look symmetrical at midline, so the amount to be used should be almost same. It is recommended to inject at the dry-wet mucosal junction when the lips became inverted in the aging process.

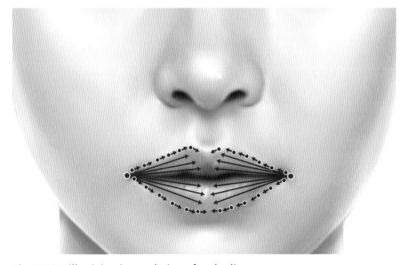

Fig. 10-2 **Filler injection technique for the lip**

Suggestive Readings

1. Braz A, Humphrey S, Weinkle S, Yee GJ, Remington BK, Lorenc ZP, et al. Lower Face: Clinical Anatomy and Regional Approaches with Injectable Fillers. Plastic and reconstructive surgery. 2015;136(5 Suppl):235s-57s.
2. Garcia de Mitchell CA, Pessa JE, Schaverien MV, Rohrich RJ. The philtrum: anatomical observations from a new perspective. Plastic and reconstructive surgery. 2008;122(6):1756-60.
3. Lee SH, Gil YC, Choi YJ, Tansatit T, Kim HJ, Hu KS. Topographic anatomy of the superior labial artery for dermal filler injection. Plastic and reconstructive surgery. 2015;135(2):445-50.
4. Penna V, Stark GB, Eisenhardt SU, Bannasch H, Iblher N. The aging lip: a comparative histological analysis of age-related changes in the upper lip complex. Plastic and reconstructive surgery. 2009;124(2):624-8.
5. Rohrich RJ, Pessa JE. The anatomy and clinical implications of perioral submuscular fat. Plastic and reconstructive surgery. 2009;124(1):266-71.

10-2 Lips

Hyun-Jo Kim, M.D., M.S., Dermatologist

10. 2. 1 Design

Several literatures describe the ideal ratio of upper lip and lower lip to be 3:5 or 9:16, but not only the proportion of the lips but also total shape of the face and facial symmetry should be considered.

10. 2. 2 Anesthesia

The lips are a very sensitive area, so regional nerve block is recommended, such as infraorbital or mental nerve block.

10. 2. 3 Technique

10. 2. 3. 1 Needle versus blunt-tip microcannula

The author prefers to use 27G or 30G needle. To make a prominent lip line, the filler should be injected along the vermilion borderline at the submucosal layer (Fig. 10-3).

To augment the lips, inject the filler at the center of the mucosa and vermilion border, and the amount of filler should be considered because of symmetry (Fig. 10-4).

10. 2. 3. 2 Filler amount

For a prominent lip line, 0.5~1 mL/lip and, for lip augmentation, 1~2 mL/lip are recommended.

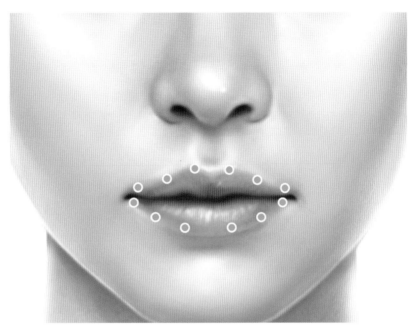

Fig. 10-3 **Filler injection technique for a prominent lip line**

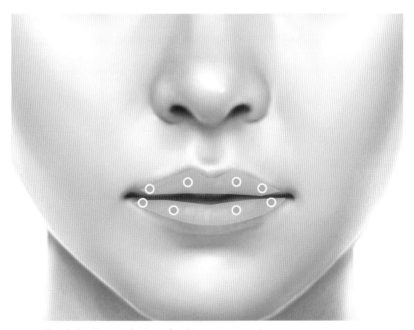

Fig. 10-4 **Filler injection technique for lip augmentation**

10. 2. 3. 3 Progress and photograph

A case of lip wrinkles and volume augmentation (Fig. 10-5).

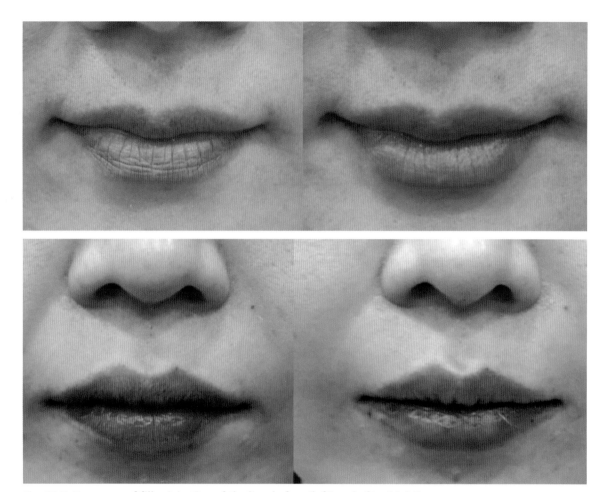

Fig. 10-5 Two cases of filler injection of the lips: before (left) and after (right)

10. 2. 3. 4 Cautions

The superior and inferior labial arteries are usually located posterior to the orbicularis oris muscle, so it is recommended not to inject the filler deeply but at the orbicularis oris muscle level or submucosal layer (Fig. 10-6).

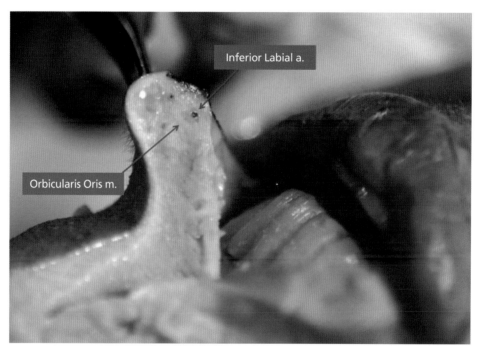

Fig. 10-6 Inferior labial artery

Suggestive Readings

1. Kim H-J, Seo KK, Lee H-K, Kim J. Clinical Anatomy of the Face for Filler and Botulinum Toxin Injection: Springer; 2016.
2. Lee SH, Lee HJ, Kim YS, Kim HJ, Hu KS. What is the difference between the inferior labial artery and the horizontal labiomental artery? Surgical and radiologic anatomy : SRA. 2015;37(8):947-53.
3. Lee SH, Lee M, Kim HJ. Anatomy-based image processing analysis of the running pattern of the perioral artery for minimally invasive surgery. The British journal of oral & maxillofacial surgery. 2014;52(8):688-92.

Lip injection at a glance

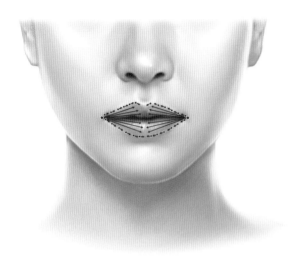 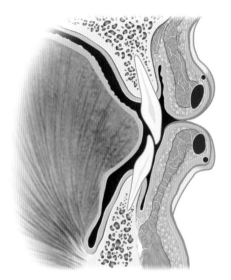

- Dr. Jeong-Jun Park (Plastic Surgeon)'s technique

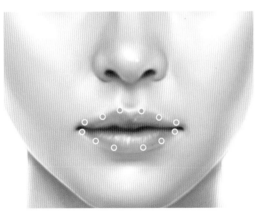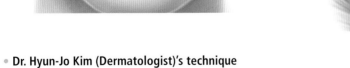 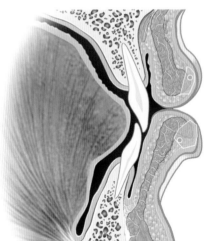

- Dr. Hyun-Jo Kim (Dermatologist)'s technique

	Dr. Park (PS)	Dr. Kim (Derma)
Needle/cannula	Dermal layer: needle 30G SubQ: cannula 23G	Needle 30G, 13 mm
Unilateral amount	Dermal layer: 0.1~0.2 mL SubQ: 0.5~1 mL	0.5~1.0 mL
Elasticity The Chaeum	Dermal layer: No. 1 SubQ: No. 1	No. 1
Anesthesia	EMLA cream application and regional nerve block	Regional nerve block
Techniques	Dermal: linear threading technique SubQ: linear threading fanning technique	Linear threading and bolus(point) injection
Layer	Dermal/subdermal layer Subcutaneous layer	Submucosal layer

*Subcutaneous layer = submucosal layer

Mentum

11-1 Mentum

Jeong-Jun Park, M.D., Ph.D., Plastic Surgeon

11. 1. 1 Considerations before injection

Western people have well-developed chins, but many Oriental people have small or short chin. Moreover, many people have bimaxillary protrusion, so it relatively appears as a small chin. In these cases, people like to close the mouth hardly by mentalis muscle hyperaction and tend to show cobble-stone appearance. Therefore, in many cases, botulinum toxin injection is combined with volumizing filler injection. The chin is important with its own shape but also very important in proportion with adjacent structures. In the frontal view, the ideal proportion would be upper 1/3, middle 1/3, and lower 1/3. However, recently, Koreans prefer slightly shorter chin and prefer to have 1:1:0.8. In the lateral view, the relationship between the nose and lips is very important. An easy method is forming what we call as Ricketts' line (Fig. 11-1). Ricketts' line is a virtual line from the nasal tip to soft tissue pogonion. The ideal relationship should be that the lips should be located at this line or 1~2 mm posterior to this line. When this line crosses the posterior of the lips, a small chin, bimaxillary prognathism, or large lips are likely present. Thus, when we perform chin augmentation, the filler amount for projection or elongation should be estimated. Usually both procedures, which are vertical elongation and anterior projection, should be performed concomitantly, but when the chin is normal or long, never perform an injection for vertical elongation.

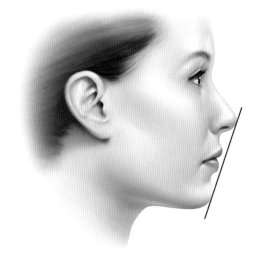

Fig. 11-1 **Ricketts' line**

11. 1. 2 Anatomical considerations

In making a harmonious and beautiful mental line, the anatomical layers should be determined. It consists of skin, superficial fat compartment, mentalis muscle, deep fat compartment, periosteum, and bone (Fig. 11-2).

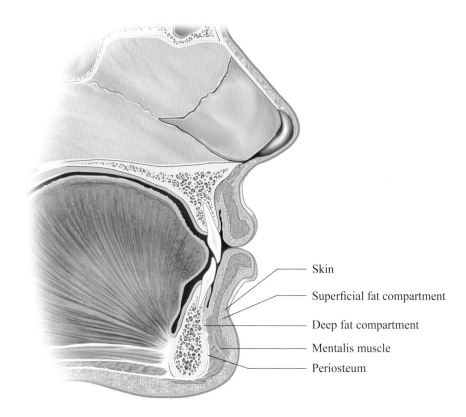

                Skin

                Superficial fat compartment

                Deep fat compartment

                Mentalis muscle

                Periosteum

Fig. 11-2 **Sagittal section of the chin**

The superficial fat compartment is known as the mental fat compartment. This connects to the labio-mandibular fat compartment laterally. Mental fat compartment has a boundary line by submental ligaments below, labio-mandibular groove laterally, and mentolabial sulcus above. The mentalis muscle is a cone-shaped muscle that originates from the incisive fossa of the lower mandible and attaches to the mental dermis layer. The lower part of the mentalis muscle tends to decussate and attaches to the dermis, so there is a space between the mandibular bone and muscle fibers. This is called submentalis fat.

It is located just below the mentalis muscle, and there is a report that it is divided bilaterally and not connected to each other. It is a relative avascular plane and needs a large amount of hard filler to be augmented. The arteries in the mental area are the mental artery from the mental foramen and inferior labial artery from the facial artery. These vessels are located at the outer layer of the injection site, but rarely, the inferior labial artery branches from the submental artery and is located at the submental triangle.

11. 1. 3 Technique

11. 1. 3. 1 Design

Draw the mentolabial sulcus and soft tissue menton. Moreover, draw midline and labio-mandibular grooves (laterally). In chin projection, the middle point is at the mentolabial sulcus and soft tissue menton, and in both elongation and projection, the point is at the soft tissue menton. To make a smooth jawline, make an entry middle point between the central point and labio-mandibular groove (Fig. 11-3).

11. 1. 3. 2 Anesthesia

EMLA cream application and local lidocaine injection at the entry point are adequate, but in highly sensitive patients, mental nerve block could be performed.

11. 1. 3. 3 Technique

11. 1. 3. 3. 1 Needle versus cannula

When volumizing the center of the chin, perforate using a needle the central entry point deep to the periosteum. Try regurgitation, and inject at the deep fat layers. For projection, needle bevel should be in the cephalic direction, and for elongation, the bevel should be in the caudal direction. When injecting not midline but on the sides, unilateral deep fat component could be augmented and might lead to asymmetry. However, when the mental crease is seen at the midline or a vessel is found through the skin, low side injection could be performed but volume should be regulated when injecting bilaterally. When the mentolabial sulcus is prominent, it might be more noticeable when there is overcorrection when injecting at the superficial fat layer, so it is recommended to inject at the deep fat layer. However, injection at the deep fat layer might induce more prominent labiomental groove by overprojection of

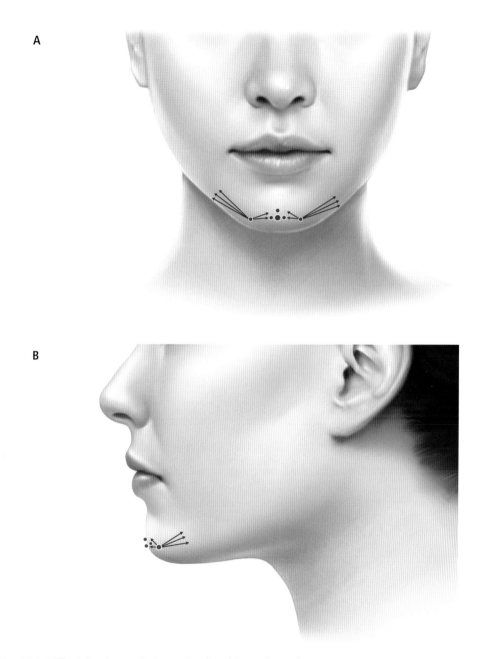

Fig. 11-3 **Filler injection techniques for the chin (A, frontal view; B, lateral view)**

the chin or irregular jawline. Thus, the superficial fat layer should also be augmented. The entry point would be lateral from midline, insert the cannula at the superficial fat layer crossing the labiomental groove, and inject slowly and retrogradely. The filler might migrate to the neck area along the platysma muscle, so protect the area with the other hand. Finally, a satisfactory result could be obtained by molding the borderline gently.

11. 1. 3. 3. 2 Filler amount
Deep fat layer: 1~3 mL
Superficial fat layer: 0.5~1 mL

11. 1. 3. 3. 3 Progress and photograph

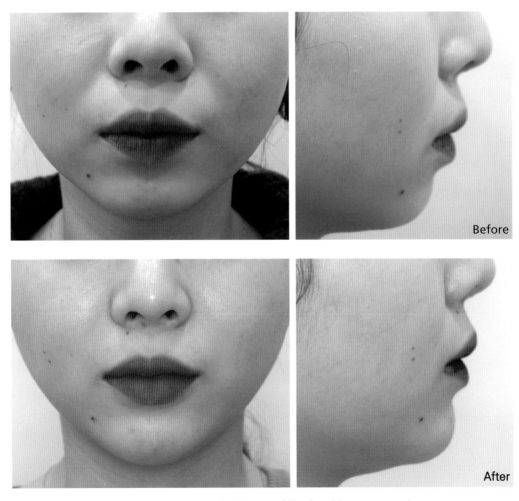

Fig. 11-4 **A 24-year-old woman is injected with 2 mL filler for chin augmentation**

Suggestive Readings

1. Braz A, Humphrey S, Weinkle S, Yee GJ, Remington BK, Lorenc ZP, et al. Lower Face: Clinical Anatomy and Regional Approaches with Injectable Fillers. Plastic and reconstructive surgery. 2015;136(5 Suppl):235s-57s.

2. Buckingham ED, Glasgold R, Kontis T, Smith SP, Jr., Dolev Y, Fitzgerald R, et al. Volume rejuvenation of the lower third, perioral, and jawline. Facial plastic surgery : FPS. 2015;31(1):70-9.

3. Gierloff M, Stohring C, Buder T, Wiltfang J. The subcutaneous fat compartments in relation to aesthetically important facial folds and rhytides. Journal of plastic, reconstructive & aesthetic surgery : JPRAS. 2012;65(10):1292-7.

4. Pilsl U, Anderhuber F. The chin and adjacent fat compartments. Dermatologic surgery : official publication for American Society for Dermatologic Surgery [et al]. 2010;36(2):214-8.

5. Rohrich RJ, Pessa JE. The anatomy and clinical implications of perioral submuscular fat. Plastic and reconstructive surgery. 2009;124(1):266-71.

11-2 Mentum

Dae-Hyun Kim, M.D., Dermatologist

11. 2. 1 Design

Chin augmentation by filler injection is a relatively easy procedure compared to augmentation of other areas, but a whole facial harmonized contour should be considered. To obtain good results, the presence of any asymmetry should be considered, and results should be predicted. Filler injection for chin projection or elongation is recommended for mild microgenia, flattened square-shaped mentum, and relative projection of the lip. Moreover, care should be taken in case of witch's chin, a condition in which the chin is extremely long, and usually, there is asymmetry; hence, the patients should be warned before injection. The procedure is as follows: draw the midline and mark soft tissue menton, pinch soft tissue to predict the results; then, draw the entry points. The entry point would be between the pogonion and menton, near the gnathion. The patient's satisfaction increases when correct chin augmentation is performed with correct labiomental groove and mental crease.

Draw the labiomental groove and mark the entry point lateral to this groove.

11. 2. 2 Anesthesia

The mental area is a relatively painless area; therefore, filler injections containing lidocaine can be performed without anesthesia. Usually, EMLA cream application is adequate.

11. 2. 3 Technique

An entry point is made lateral to the labiomental groove using a needle, and a relative soft filler injection of 0.5 mL/side is performed at the subcutaneous layer using a cannula. When there is asymmetry, it is useful to correct at the subcutaneous layer. It is recommended not to inject more than 1 mL on each side because it might result in irregular contour.

It is important to inject at the deep layer in chin projection or elongation. Usually, the filler is injected under the mentalis muscle or supraperiosteal layer using a needle. One hand should hold the entry point area, and the filler is injected with the other hand. When the needle tip is attached to the bone, re-adjust the position so that the needle is placed between the mandibular bone and mentalis muscle. The required shape can be obtained by molding after injection, but it is better to the make the shape during injection; therefore, we pinch the area with the non-injecting hand. The filler does not tend to migrate when it is injected at the deep layer, but a large amount of the filler is required. It is important to prevent asymmetry and formation of an irregular borderline. When the injection is performed at a deep-seated site, usually, 1~2 mL of filler is used. However, when a large volume is injected, discomfort or pain might be experienced after the procedure. When there is an irregular borderline, molding should be performed.

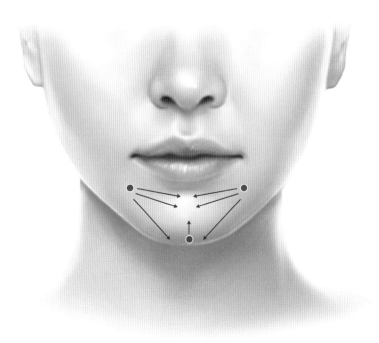

Fig. 11-5 Technique

11. 2. 4 Filler amount

Inject 1~2 mL of the filler at the supraperiosteal or deep fat layer to augment the mentum and 0.5~1 mL/side at the superficial fat layer of the labiomental groove and mentum.

11. 2. 5 Progress and photograph

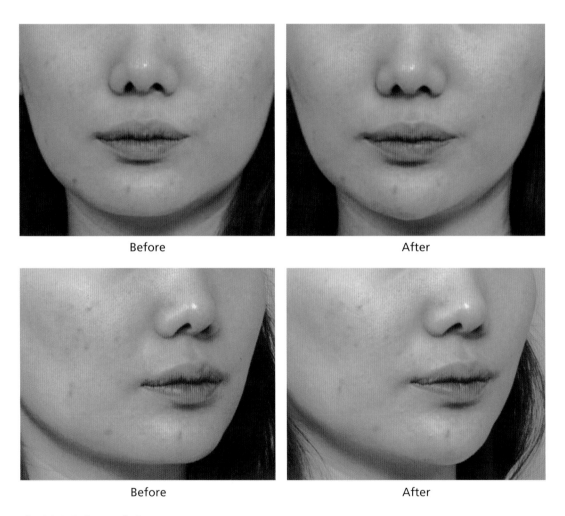

Before

After

Before

After

Fig. 11-6 **Before and after**

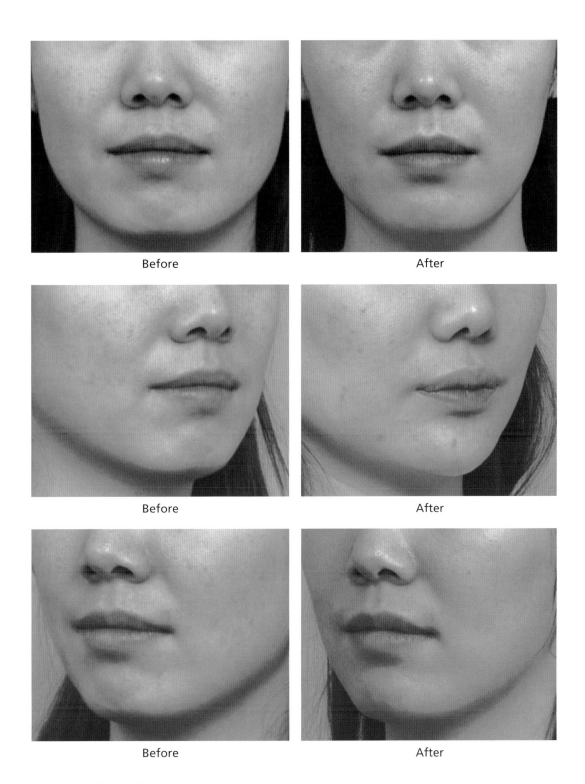

Before

After

Before

After

Before

After

Fig. 11-7 **Before and after**

Suggestive Readings

1. Vanaman Wilson MJ, Jones IT, Butterwick K, Fabi SG. Role of Nonsurgical Chin Augmentation in Full Face Rejuvenation: A Review and Our Experience. Dermatologic surgery : official publication for American Society for Dermatologic Surgery [et al]. 2018;44(7):985-93.
2. de Maio M, Wu WTL, Goodman GJ, Monheit G. Facial Assessment and Injection Guide for Botulinum Toxin and Injectable Hyaluronic Acid Fillers: Focus on the Lower Face. Plastic and reconstructive surgery. 2017;140(3):393e-404e.
3. Kim H-J, Seo KK, Lee H-K, Kim J. Clinical Anatomy of the Face for Filler and Botulinum Toxin Injection: Springer; 2016.

Chin augmentation at a glance

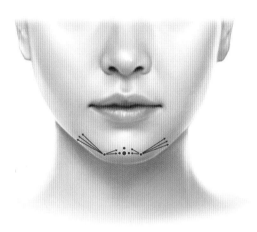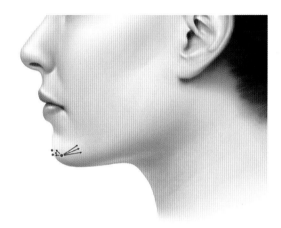

- **Dr. Jeong-Jun Park (Plastic Surgeon)'s technique**

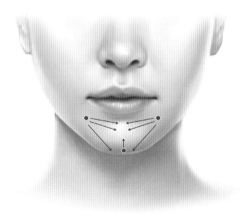

- **Dr. Dae-Hyun Kim (Dermatologist)'s technique**

	Dr. Park (PS)	Dr. Kim (Derma)
Needle/cannula	Deep: needle 27G, SubQ: cannula 23G	Deep: needle 27G, SubQ: cannula 25G
Unilateral amount	Deep: 1~3mL, SubQ: 0.5~1 mL	Deep: 1~2 mL, SubQ: 0.5~1 mL
Elasticity The Chaeum	Deep: No.3, SubQ: No.2	Deep: No.3, SubQ: No.1 or No.2
Anesthesia	EMLA cream application and local lidocaine injection	EMLA cream application
Techniques	Deep: Bolus, SubQ: linear threading fanning technique	Deep: Bolus, SubQ: linear threading fanning technique
Layer	Deep: supraperiosteal layer, SubQ: subcutaneous layer	Deep: supraperiosteal layer, SubQ: subcutaneous layer

Upper eyelids (sunken eyelids)

12-1 Sunken upper eyelid

Yong-Woo Lee, M.D., M.B.A., Plastic Surgeon

12. 1. 1 Design

Recommended injection site

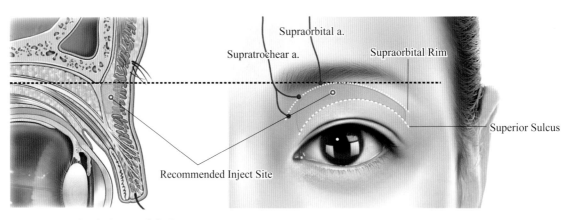

Fig. 12-1 Sagittal view and design

12. 1. 2 Anesthesia

Local lidocaine injection is performed at the entry point. Regional nerve block could be performed, but extensive anesthesia is not recommended because the layers can be easily dehisced with low resistance.

12. 1. 3 Technique

12. 1. 3. 1 Needle versus cannula

A 23G 3.2 cm needle is used at the lateral side, and all areas are augmented at once.

12. 1. 3. 2 Filler amount

Less than 0.5 mL of filler is used unilaterally. When an additional amount is needed, it is recommended to perform the injection after 2 weeks.

12. 1. 3. 3 Cautions

Do not overcorrect at once. It is recommended to inject insufficiently and consider additional injections. It is very important not to perforate the orbital septum but inject as deepest as possible because the eyes might appear bulged after closing.

12. 1. 3. 4 Complications and management

Periorbital bruising is the most common complication. The filler should be injected gently because of high vascularity and serious complications such as blindness. Skin necrosis does not develop even though it is very near the eye. It is a highly vascularized area, but the vessels are small in diameter and might tear. However, this does not cause embolism. The problem might occur when injection is performed behind the orbital septum. When injection is performed behind the orbital septum, bleeding might occur, and adjacent structures are compressed and might lead to fibrosis of the levator palpebrae superioris muscle. Therefore, the filler should be injected in front of the orbital septum.

Suggestive Readings

1.   Liew S, Nguyen DQ. Nonsurgical volumetric upper periorbital rejuvenation: a plastic surgeon's perspective. Aesthetic plastic surgery. 2011;35(3):319-25.
2.   Lin TM, Lin TY, Chou CK, Lai CS, Lin SD. Application of microautologous fat transplantation in the correction of sunken upper eyelid. Plastic and reconstructive surgery Global open. 2014;2(11):e259.
3.   Park S, Kim B, Shin Y. Correction of superior sulcus deformity with orbital fat anatomic repositioning and fat graft applied to retro-orbicularis oculi fat for Asian eyelids. Aesthetic plastic surgery. 2011;35(2):162-70.

12-2 Sunken upper eyelid

Gi-Woong Hong, M.D., Ph.D., Plastic Surgeon

12. 2. 1 Considerations before injection

People with congenital or acquired sunken eyelids look old, tired, or sleepy. Their causes are genetic, orbital fat volume decrease in the aging process, or excessive fat removal by previous blepharoplasty. Oriental people have relatively weak levator palpebrae superioris muscle, which are not attached to the dermis, and the consequences of having a single fold. Skin and fats are likely to droop, and the orbital rim area appears swollen and bulging. In contrast, the volume of the orbital septal fat is likely to decrease, the power of levator palpebrae superioris muscle is likely to weaken, and drooping skin also develops. All these phenomena result in typical sunken upper eyelids. Sunken upper eyelids lead to fatigue appearance, blepharoptosis, and uncertain double folds. This means that augmenting the sunken portion, which is under the orbital rim and upper supratarsal lid crease, can improve the sleepy and distinct eye appearance and prominent double folds.

12. 2. 2 Technique

It is very important to inject soft filler at the sunken upper eyelids by retrograde linear threading small volume technique and with open eyes and in a sitting position. Injecting at the OOM and inside the orbital septum would increase the risk of bleeding. This space is also at risk for hemostasis during bleeding and hematoma, which could damage the septum. The recommended layer would be the preseptal space outside the orbital septum along theorbital rim margin. The supratrochlear and supraorbital arteries are located at the medial orbital rim area, and inside the orbit, they anastomosed with the central retinal artery, so care should be taken when injection is performed, and it is recommended to use a cannula (Fig. 12-2).

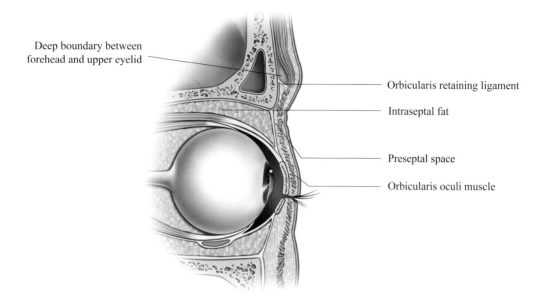

Deep boundary between
forehead and upper eyelid

Orbicularis retaining ligament

Intraseptal fat

Preseptal space

Orbicularis oculi muscle

Fig. 12-2 Preseptal space of upper eyelid

The entry point would be at the vertical line on the lateral canthus. Perforate the orbital rim area until the orbital rim bone using a cannula, and locate the supraperiosteal layer. There is less fatty tissue deeper than the OOM, so try to inject near the orbital septum evenly with a soft filler (Fig. 12-3). It is important to check whether there are any irregularities when the eyes are closed, and when there is overcorrection, the filler would migrate to eyelids, so undercorrection is recommended (Fig. 12-4). After injection, if there is any depressed or prominent border, fill it with a soft filler at the subdermal layer, but since the eyelids are very thin, having no lumps should be considered (Fig. 12-5). In case of blepharoptosis or exophthalmos, a good result could not be expected, and if there is any previous scar, the filler could not be evenly injected.

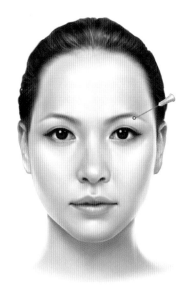

Injection at the entry point:
Vertical line on the lateral canthus around the lower margin of the superior orbital rim – mainly the medial parts of the periorbital rim under the brow to avoid the supraorbital and supratrochlear main vessel branches above the supratarsal lid crease and under the orbicularis retaining ligament.

Injection technique:
- vertical sitting position
- voluntarily opened eyes
- retrograde linear threading small volume injection
- very slow release

Fig. 12-3 Supraorbital hollowness: injection techniques

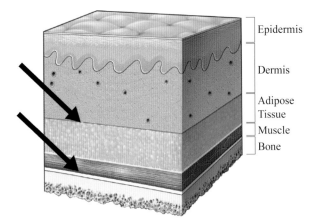

Injection plane
- Supraperiosteal and submuscular injection around the orbital rim over the orbital septum – Restylane Vital or Vital Light 0.3~0.5 mL for each area: 30G cannula
- Submuscular injection into the sub-orbicularis oculi fat (SOOF) for brow augmentation – Restylane Lidocaine 0.3~0.5 mL for each area: 30G cannula
- Subdermal injection of Restylane Vital Light to even the surface and remove unnecessary multiple eyelid lines – Restylane Vital Light 0.1~0.2 mL for each area: 33G nanoneedle

Fig. 12-4 Supraorbital hollowness: injection plane and products

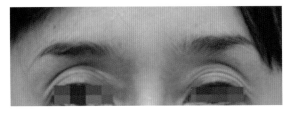 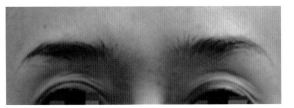

Fig. 12-5 Sunken upper eyelids: before and after

Suggestive Readings

1. Cohen JL, Brown MR. Anatomic considerations for soft tissue augmentation of the face. Journal of drugs in dermatology : JDD. 2009;8(1):13-6.
2. Lin TM, Lin TY, Chou CK, Lai CS, Lin SD. Application of microautologous fat transplantation in the correction of sunken upper eyelid. Plastic and reconstructive surgery Global open. 2014;2(11):e259.
3. Park SH, Sun HJ, Choi KS. Sudden unilateral visual loss after autologous fat injection into the nasolabial fold. Clinical ophthalmology (Auckland, NZ). 2008;2(3):679-83.
4. Salati SA. Complications of Dermal Filling. Online J Health Allied Scs. 2011;10(3):9

12-3 Sunken upper eyelid

Hyun-Jo Kim, M.D., M.S., Dermatologist

12. 3. 1 Design

The puncture point is shown in Fig. 12-6. Three to six points are made.

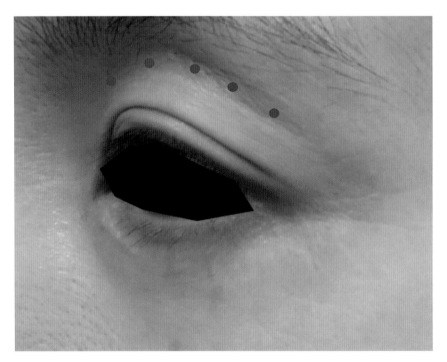

Fig. 12-6 Injection point in correction of sunken upper eyelids

12. 3. 2 Anesthesia

EMLA cream application is sufficient.

12. 3. 3 Techniques

12. 3. 3. 1 Needle versus blunt-tip microcannula

The author prefers a 33G needle because a small amount of filler is used. It is recommended not to perforate the orbital septum and inject at the ROOF level (Fig. 12-7).

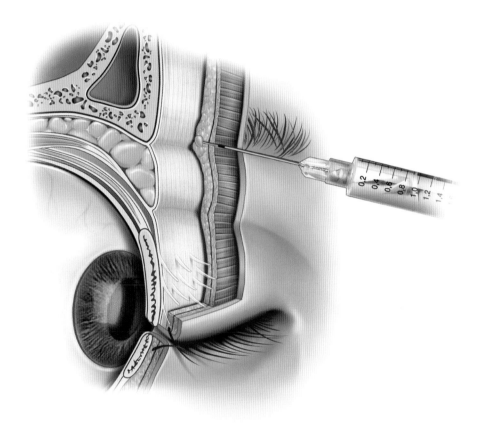

Fig. 12-7 **Filler injection site to correct sunken upper eyelids**

By palpating the superior orbital rim, insert the needle. After feeling for the superior orbital rim, move the tip slightly backward, and inject at the ROOF level by bolus technique. It is convenient to inject at the medial side first and then the lateral side (Figs. 12-8 and 12-9).

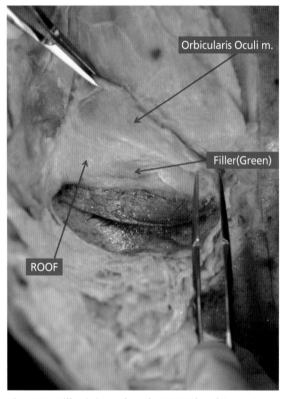

Fig. 12-8 **Filler injected at the ROOF level (green)**

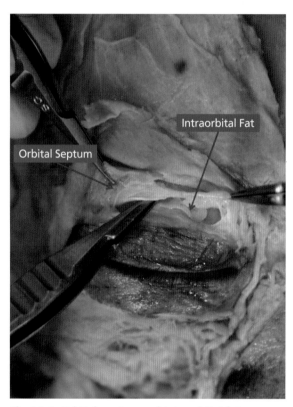

Fig. 12-9 **Orbital septum and intraorbital fat**

12. 3. 3. 2 Filler amount

The filler amount is 0.2~0.4 mL unilaterally.

12. 3. 3. 3 Progress and photograph

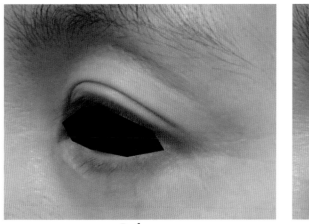 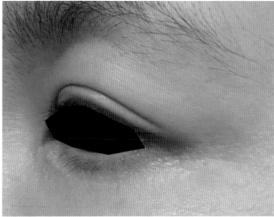

Before   After

Fig. 12-10 **Sunken upper eyelids: before and after**

12. 3. 3. 4 Cautions

A small amount of filler is very effective, but care should be taken because it might result in a sleepy or tired appearance when there is overcorrection.

It is recommended to determine the pathways of the supraorbital, supratrochlear, and superior medial palpebral arteries to avoid vascular compromise (Fig. 12-11).

It is important not to perforate the orbital septum because complications such as hematoma or disturbance of eyeball movement might develop.

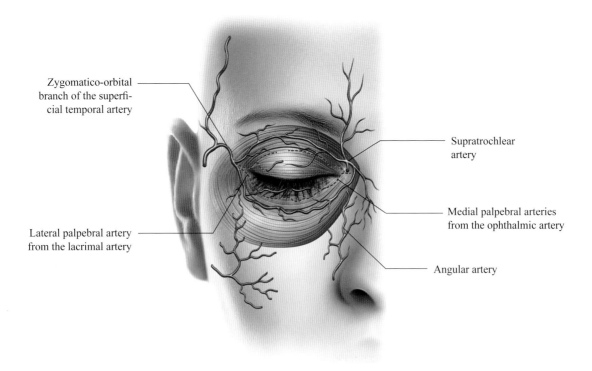

Zygomatico-orbital branch of the superficial temporal artery

Supratrochlear artery

Lateral palpebral artery from the lacrimal artery

Medial palpebral arteries from the ophthalmic artery

Angular artery

Fig. 12-11 Periorbital arteries in sunken upper eyelid correction

Suggestive Readings

1. Hwang SH, Hwang K, Jin S, Kim DJ. Location and nature of retro-orbicularis oculus fat and suborbicularis oculi fat. The Journal of craniofacial surgery. 2007;18(2):387-90.
2. Kim H-J, Seo KK, Lee H-K, Kim J. Clinical Anatomy of the Face for Filler and Botulinum Toxin Injection: Springer; 2016.
3. Looi AL, Yong KL. "Walk the Rim, Feel the Bone" Technique in Superior Sulcus Filling. Plastic and reconstructive surgery Global open. 2015;3(12):e592.

Sunken upper eyelid correction at a glance

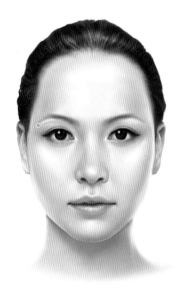
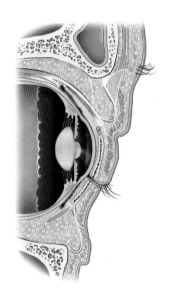

- **Dr. Yong-Woo Lee (Plastic Surgeon)'s technique**

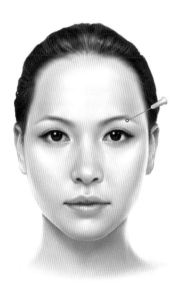
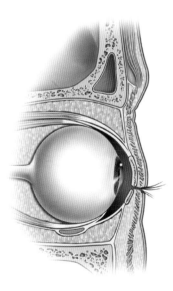

- **Dr. Gi-Woong Hong (Plastic Surgeon)'s technique**

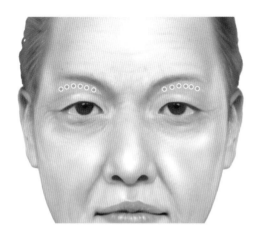
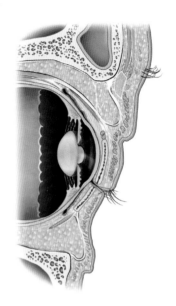

● **Dr. Hyun-Jo Kim (Dermatologist)'s technique**

	Dr. Lee (PS)	Dr. Hong (PS)	Dr. Kim (Derma)
Needle/cannula	Needle 23G, 3.2 cm	Cannula 30G	Needle 33G
Unilateral amount	Approximately 0.5 mL	0.3~0.5 mL	0.2~0.4 mL
Elasticity The Chaeum	No.2	No.1	No.1
Anesthesia	Local lidocaine injection	EMLA cream application and local lidocaine injection at the entry point	EMLA cream application
Techniques	Bolus technique	Retrograde linear threading small volume injection technique	Linear threading and bolus technique
Layer	Just below the supraorbital rim. Not to inject superficially because it might result in an irregular shape.	Space between the OOM and orbital septum Subdermal layer to obtain a smooth contour	ROOF level

Infraorbital hollowness

13-1 Infraorbital groove and hollowness

Dr. Choon-Shik Youn, M.D., Dermatologist

13. 1. 1 Tear trough–palpebromalar groove pathophysiology

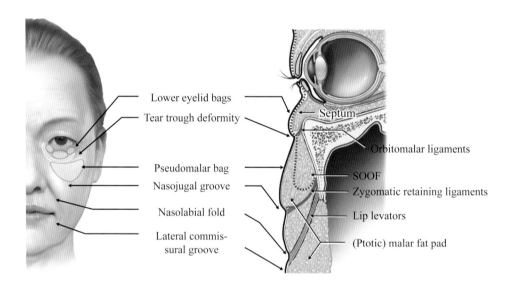

Lower eyelid bags
Tear trough deformity
Pseudomalar bag
Nasojugal groove
Nasolabial fold
Lateral commissural groove

Septum
Orbitomalar ligaments
SOOF
Zygomatic retaining ligaments
Lip levators
(Ptotic) malar fat pad

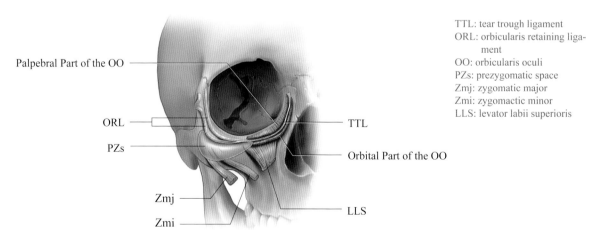

Palpebral Part of the OO
ORL
PZs
Zmj
Zmi

TTL
Orbital Part of the OO
LLS

TTL: tear trough ligament
ORL: orbicularis retaining liga-
      ment
OO: orbicularis oculi
PZs: prezygomatic space
Zmj: zygomatic major
Zmi: zygomactic minor
LLS: levator labii superioris

Fig. 13-1 Midface anatomy: Retaining ligament

1) Tear trough–palpebromalar groove develops by pulling the tear trough and orbitomalar ligaments

2) Loss of structural support

- Tear trough/palpebromalar groove tends to be more prominent in eye-bag ptosis above the tear trough/orbitomalar groove and there are loss of volume and downward descent of the superficial fat and deep fat under the groove.

- Tear trough/palpebromalar groove tends to be more prominent due to maxillary bone absorption.

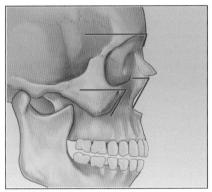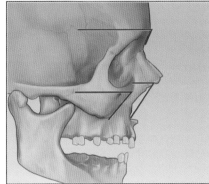

Fig. 13-2 **Volume loss: Bone**

3) Differences between tear trough–palpebromalar groove on the upper and lower sides

- The upper side has a thin skin and lacks fat tissue, but the lower side has thicker skin and more abundant fat tissues.

13. 1. 2 Midcheek groove pathophysiology

1) It occurs at the zygomatic cutaneous ligament.

2) Groove is deepened by continuous movement of the lip elevator muscles.

3) Midcheek groove is deepened by volume loss of SOOF, which is located above the zygomatic cutaneous ligament, and lateral part of the deep medial cheek fat (DMCF), which is located below the zygomatic cutaneous ligament.

4) Bone absorption: midcheek groove is deepened by maxillary bone absorption.

5) Midcheek groove is deepened by malar mound ptosis, which develops by loosening of the antero-medial cheek soft tissue retaining ligament.

13. 1. 3 Surface anatomy

13. 1. 3. 1 Tear trough and palpebromalar groove

It is difficult to define the tear trough because it has different descriptions in literatures. Generally, Nicholas et al. described the tear trough as located from the medial canthus to midpupillary line and palpebromalar groove as from the midpupillary line to lateral canthus, and the author also believes this conceptualization is appropriate.

13. 1. 3. 2 Midcheek groove

It is also called as "Indian band" and has the same location as the zygomatic cutaneous ligament.

There are tear trough and orbitomalar ligaments beneath the tear trough and palpebromalar groove, and these ligaments are continuous and true retaining ligaments. The zygomatic cutaneous ligament is a discontinuous structure and a false retaining ligament at the anteromedial cheek area. Thus, the midcheek groove does not appear clinically.

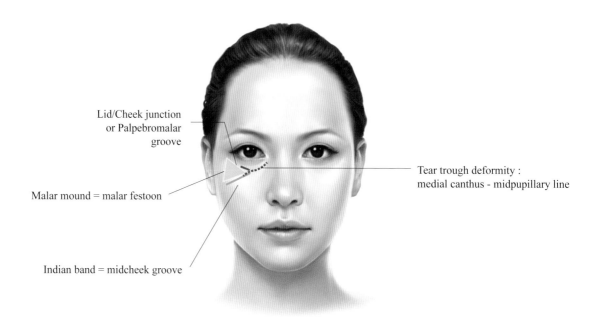

Fig. 13-3 Surface anatomy: tear trough, palpebromalar groove, and midcheek groove

13. 1. 4 Design

13. 1. 4. 1 Tear trough and palpebromalar groove

Left face: five areas to check for degree of hollowness

Right face: actual injection at four areas (Fig. 13-4)

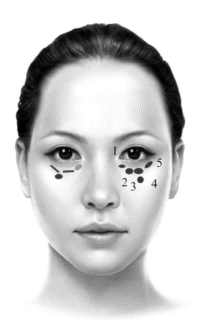

Fig. 13-4 Injection area (zones 1–5) and technique

13. 1. 4. 2 Midcheek groove

Draw a virtual line starting from the tear trough and oblique line along the Indian band, and draw across the vertical line of the midpupillary line and make the cross point as the central point to be injected (Fig. 13-5).

13. 1. 5 Anesthesia

13. 1. 5. 1 Tear trough and palpebromalar groove

This area is relatively not painful, so the author applies EMLA cream in most cases, and when other

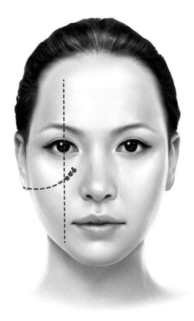

Fig. 13-5 Injection area of midcheek groove

procedures (syringoma, pretarsal fullness, and anteromedial cheek augmentation) should be performed together, infraorbital nerve block might be considered.

13. 1. 5. 2 Midcheek groove

Regional nerve block is preferred when deep injection at the submuscular level is performed, and EMLA cream application when superficial injection at the subdermal level is performed.

13. 1. 6 Technique

13. 1. 6. 1 Tear trough and palpebromalar groove

Inject using the linear threading technique.

13. 1. 6. 1. 1 Injection depth (Fig. 13-6)

Inject at the submuscular or supraperiosteal level.

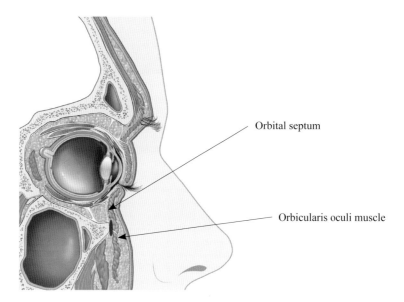

Fig. 13-6 **Injection depth**

To correct a palpebromalar groove, injection is performed at the SOOF level. However, there is less SOOF at the tear trough level, which is under the OOM, so injecting at the tear trough means not injecting at the SOOF but actually inside the OOM or between the bone and OOM or between the skin and OOM.

* Superficial (subdermal) injection technique

When correcting a tear trough deformity or palpebromalar groove, injecting deeply (submuscular level) could prevent lumps, swelling, and discoloration. However, there are some wrinkles that are not covered by deep injection. In this case, it is better to inject at the subdermal layer additionally with low-elasticity soft filler.

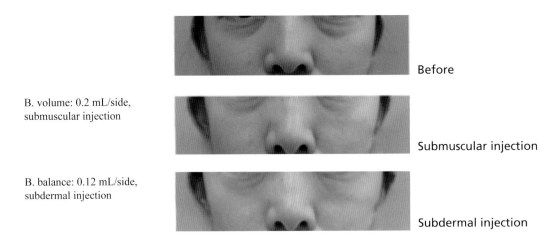

B. volume: 0.2 mL/side,
submuscular injection

Before

Submuscular injection

B. balance: 0.12 mL/side,
subdermal injection

Subdermal injection

Fig. 13-7 **Superficial injection: Subdermal**

13. 1. 6. 1. 2 Needle versus cannula

To inject precisely, it is recommended to use a needle, but it would cause more bruising. In contrast, to prevent bruising, it is better to use a cannula, but it is less precise.

Needle	Blunt Cannula
More bruise	Less bruise
More edema	Less edema
More precise	Less precise

13. 1. 6. 1. 3 Filler amount

The filler amount is 0.4~0.8 mL/side.

13. 1. 6. 1. 4 Molding

When injecting at the tear trough or palpebromalar groove, the filler is likely to aggregate, so the patient is recommended to visit within 1 week and massage the area to spread the filler.

There is greater improvement after molding.

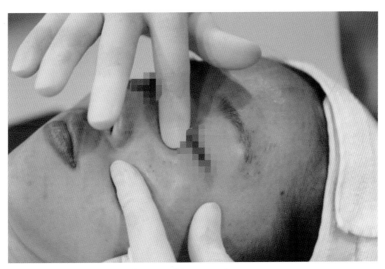

Fig. 13-8 **Follow-up molding within 1 week**

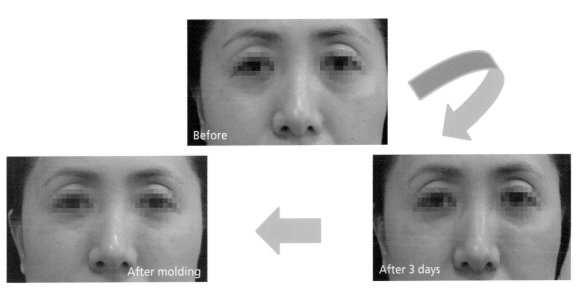

Fig. 13-9 **Follow-up molding within 1 week**

13. 1. 6. 1. 5 Progress and photograph

Tear trough deformity and palpebromalar groove can be classified into three types.

1. Tear trough & Palpebromalar groove only

2. Tear trough & Palpebromalar + Mild fat bulging

3. Tear trough & Palpebromalar + Malar retraction

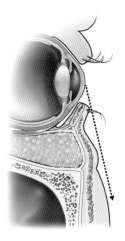 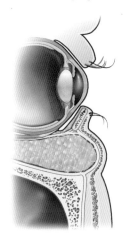 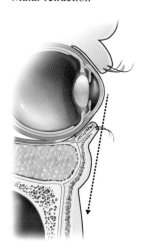

Fig. 13-10 Tear trough and palpebromalar groove: classification

Type 1. Tear trough and palpebromalar groove only

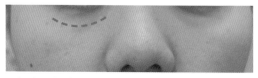

Submuscular level: Linear thread injection Belotero balance 0.07 mL *3

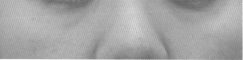 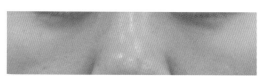

Before   4 weeks after

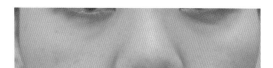 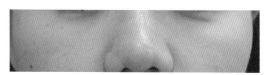

Before   24 weeks after

Fig. 13-11 Tear trough and palpebromalar groove only

Type 2. Tear trough and palpebromalar groove + mild fat bulging

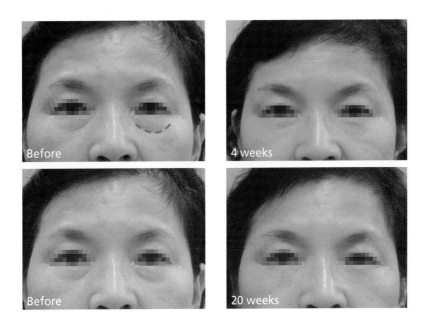

Fig. 13-12 Tear trough and palpebromalar groove + mild fat bulging

Belotero balance/deep injection/linear thread 0.15 mL*2

It is much improved by just correction of tear trough and palpebromalar groove without fat removal

Type 3. Tear trough and palpebromalar groove + malar retraction

When malar retraction is performed simultaneously, correction should be performed concomitantly to obtain appropriate convexity when a vertical line is drawn from the midpupillary line.

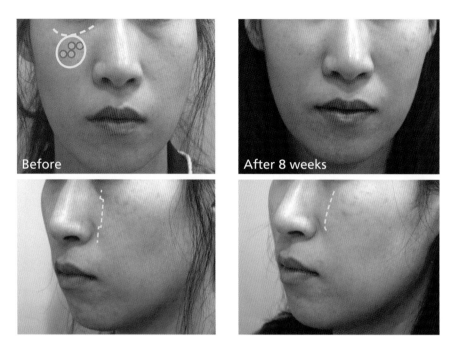

Fig. 13-13 Tear trough + Malar retraction
Yvoire Classic, 0.3 mL/side; volume, 1 mL/side

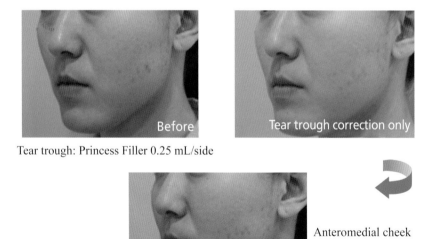

Tear trough: Princess Filler 0.25 mL/side

Anteromedial cheek
Princess Volume 0.5 mL/side

Fig. 13-14 Tear trough versus tear trough + anteromedial cheek augmentation

Smooth convexity is observed in tear trough and anteromedial cheek augmentation compared to that in tear trough correction only.

13. 1. 6. 1. 6 Longevity

Longevity depends on the filler product type but is usually 1~2 years.

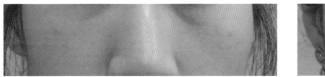 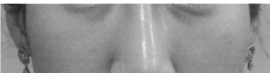

Before   20 months

Fig. 13-15 Longevity

After 20 months filler injection, still corrected tear trough

* This is a case of injected filler at the tear trough and anteromedial cheek and nasolabial fold together. One year after injection, it can be noticed that the filler still remains at the tear trough area. One of the factors of filler longevity is injected area movements, so if there is less movement in the area, the filler has lasts longer.

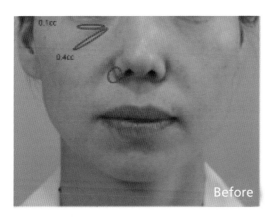 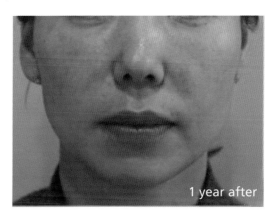

Fig. 13-16 Longevity depends on location

Elravie Deep Line – tear trough + anteromedial cheek: 0.5 mL/side (needle)

Nasolabial fold: 0.45 mL/side (needle)

13. 1. 6. 1. 7 Cautions

- A 30G or 31G needle is recommended because of easy bruising.

- The angular artery and vein are located along the tear trough, so care should be taken to prevent vascular compromise.

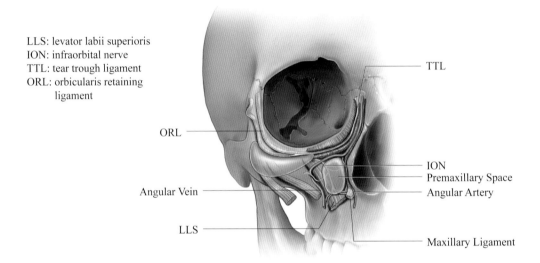

LLS: levator labii superioris
ION: infraorbital nerve
TTL: tear trough ligament
ORL: orbicularis retaining
　　　ligament

TTL

ORL

ION
Premaxillary Space
Angular Artery

Angular Vein

LLS

Maxillary Ligament

Fig. 13-17 Angular vein and artery

- Injection should be performed at the sitting position because injection above the tear trough would aggravate eye-bag bulging.

13. 1. 6. 1. 8 Complications and management

- Tyndall effect: the filler has a bluish color when injected superficially. It should be injected under the muscle when the skin is thin.

- Nodule: when one site is overinjected, it can be seen as aggregated like a nodule. The filler should be spread by molding, or diluted hyaluronidase can be injected minimally.

13. 1. 6. 2 Midcheek groove

13. 1. 6. 2. 1 Injection depth

Subdermal injection or subdermal + supraperiosteal layer injection

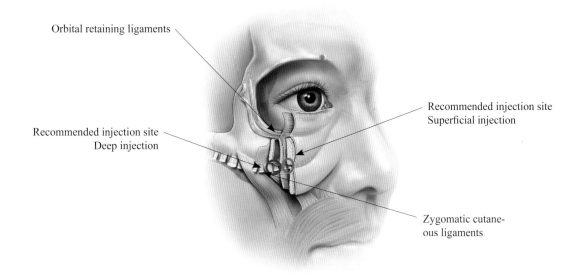

Fig. 13-18 Injection depth

- When there is a shallow groove, subdermal injection is performed. When it is deep, injection is performed at the subdermal and supraperiosteal layers (sandwich technique).

When injecting filler at the supraperiosteal layer of the midcheek groove, it is likely to be injected between the SOOF, which is located above the zygomatic cutaneous ligament, and DMCF, which is located under the ligament, but since the ligament loosens in the aging process, it is likely to be injected at the DMCF.

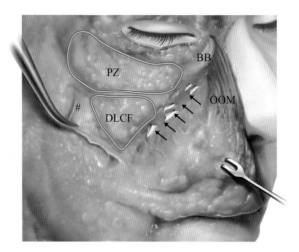

Fig. 13-19 **Layer 4: SOOF and DMCF (lateral part); PZ, prezygomatic space; BB, bare bone**

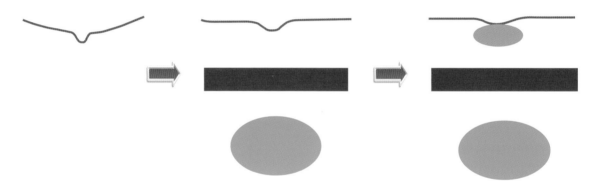

Fig. 13-20 **Sandwich technique**

Fig. 13-21 shows the deep fat component after the OOM is flipped over. The author injects at different depths according to the thickness of soft tissue. When the soft tissue is thick, the filler is injected at the upper part of deep fat,and when the soft tissue is thin, the filler is injected at the lower part of deep fat (Fig. 13-22).

13. 1. 6. 2. 2 Filler amount

The filler amount depends on the depth but is usually 0.5~1.5 mL/side

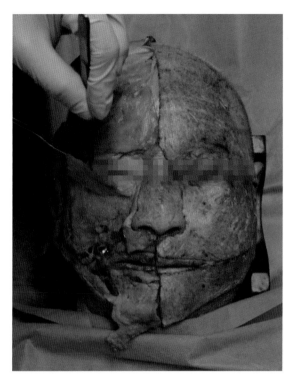 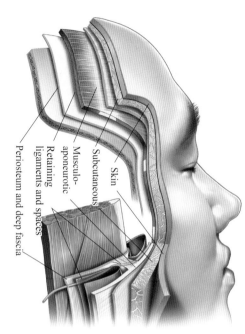

Skin
Subcutaneous
Musculo-
aponeurotic
Retaining
ligaments and spaces
Periosteum and deep fascia

Fig. 13-21 Layer 4

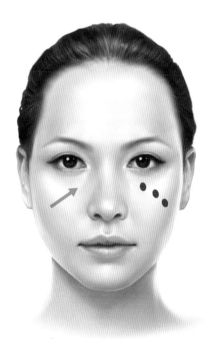

Fig. 13-22 Technique

Cannula: linear threading technique/submuscular (green color)
Needle: vertical injection technique/subcutaneous (red color)

13. 1. 6. 2. 3 Progress and photograph

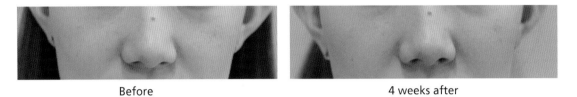

Before   4 weeks after

Fig. 13-23 Midcheek groove before and after 4 weeks
Perlane: 1 mL/side

The midcheek groove soft tissue is thin in this case, so it could be augmented with a small amount.

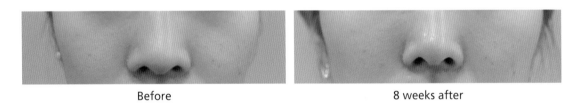

Before   8 weeks after

Fig. 13-24 Midcheek groove before and after 8 weeks
Belotero volume: 0.5 mL/side

To correct midcheek groove and tear trough simultaneously, smooth contour convexity of the midface can be obtained.

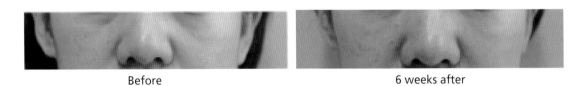

Before   6 weeks after

Fig. 13-25 Midcheek groove + tear trough
Midcheek groove – Cutegel Max: right, 1.3 mL; left, 1.2 mL
Tear trough – Cutegel: 0.25 mL/side
Cutegel Aqua: 0.25 mL/side

Even though there are prominent eyebags, it would provide better convexity by correcting tear trough and midcheek groove.

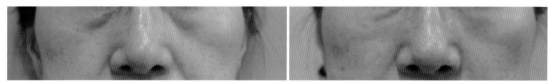

Fig. 13-26 **Midcheek groove + tear trough + eyebags**

13. 1. 6. 2. 4 Cautions

When the groove is deep, it is recommended not to correct at once because the filler might spread to adjacent regions and the groove tends to look deeper. Therefore, first correct 60~70%, and when the tissues are loosened, correct the rest.

13. 1. 6. 2. 5 Complications and management

When midcheek groove is corrected using a needle, inject at the subdermal or supraperiosteal layer because of the facial artery detour branch and facial vein tend to run nearby.

13-2 Infraorbital groove and hollowness

Hyun-Jo Kim, M.D., M.S., Dermatologist

13. 2. 1 Infraorbital hollowness: Tear trough and palpebromalar groove

13. 2. 1. 1 Design

The pathophysiology has multiple causes, but the main cause is skin change during the aging process of the orbicularis retaining ligament (Fig. 13-27).

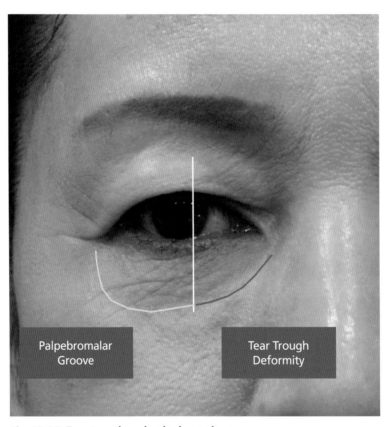

Palpebromalar Groove

Tear Trough Deformity

Fig. 13-27 Tear trough and palpebromalar groove

The orbicularis retaining ligament is divided into the vertical line from the medial pupillary line, tear trough ligament (TTL) medially, and lateral orbicularis retaining ligament (Fig. 13-28).

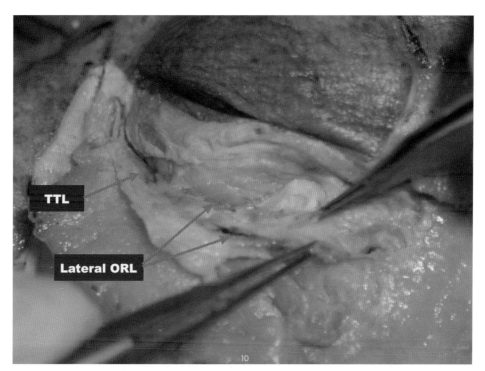

Fig. 13-28 **Tear Trough Ligament and Lateral Orbicularis Retaining Ligament**

The TTL is one of the causes of tear trough deformity, and lateral orbicularis retaining ligament laxity in the aging process causes palpebromalar groove. Thus, design at the TTL and depressed area of the lateral orbicularis retaining ligament.

13. 2. 1. 2 Anesthesia

Usually, EMLA cream application is adequate.

13. 2. 1. 3 Technique

13. 2. 1. 3. 1 Needle versus blunt-tip microcannula

In case of TTL hardly attaching to the skin (Fig. 13-29), there should be a procedure of release of TTL at the subcutaneous layer (retinacula cutis) using a microcannula (Fig. 13-30), and therefore, a blunt-tip microcannula is needed. However, in case of tear trough not holding the skin tightly, injecting the filler superficial to the OOM using a 33G needle would be an effective correction technique (Fig. 13-31).

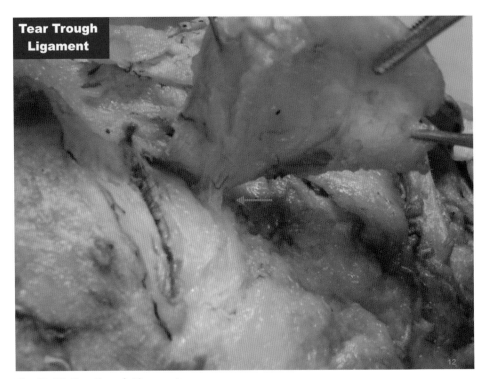

Fig. 13-29 Tear Trough Ligament

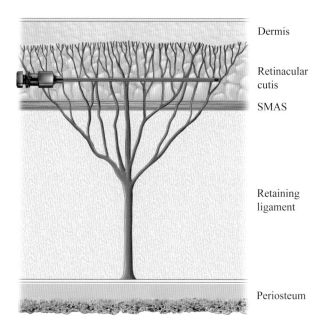

Dermis

Retinacular cutis

SMAS

Retaining ligament

Periosteum

Fig. 13-30 Tear trough ligament release using a cannula

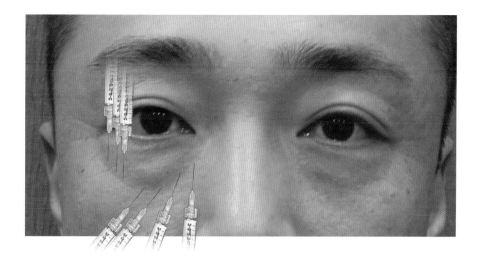

Fig. 13-31 Injection technique using a needle to correct tear trough deformity and palpebromalar groove

13. 2. 1. 3. 2 Filler amount

A small amount is effective. For tear trough deformity correction, 0.2~0.5 mL/side and for correction of palpebromalar groove, 0.2~0.5 mL/side could be sufficient.

13. 2. 1. 3. 3 Progress and photograph

A case of correcting tear trough deformity and palpebromalar groove using a 33G needle (Fig. 13-32).

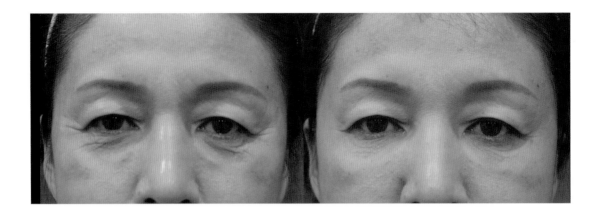

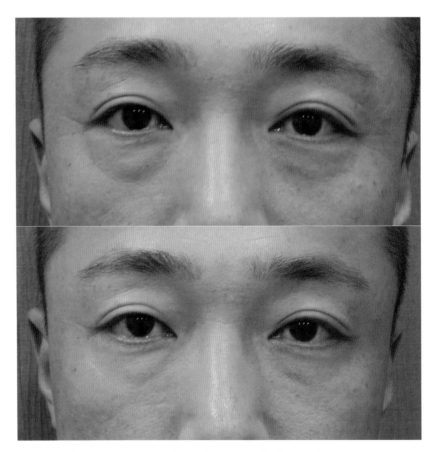

Fig. 13-32 **Tear trough deformity and palpebromalar groove: before and after**

13. 2. 1. 3. 4 Cautions

When the TTL is holding the skin tightly, it is recommended to release the ligament first; otherwise, the filler would be injected on the upper or lower part of the ligament, which could lead to unsatisfactory results.

The angular artery and vein run in a similar location to the tear trough deformity, so it is important to aspirate before injection and try to palpate for arterial pulsation to avoid vascular complications (Fig. 13-33).

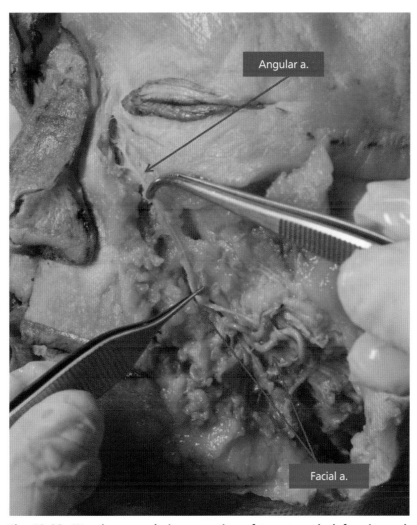

Fig. 13-33 Warning vessels in correction of tear trough deformity and palpebromalar groove

13. 2. 2 Midcheek groove and nasojugal groove

13. 2. 2. 1 Design

It should be called midcheek and nasojugal grooves and is also called Indian band, but it is a racist word and should not be used.

Usually, when zygomatic cutaneous ligament attaches to the skin tightly and usually combines with volume loss of the anteromedial cheek, it is recommended to correct them together (Fig. 13-34).

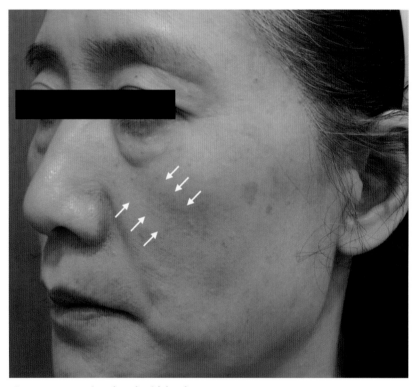

Fig. 13-34 Nasojugal and midcheek grooves

13. 2. 2. 2 Anesthesia

Usually, the ligament should be released and severe pain would occur, so infraorbital nerve regional block is recommended.

13. 2. 2. 3 Technique

13. 2. 2. 3. 1 Needle versus blunt-tip microcannula

The author uses a blunt-tip microcannula because the zygomatic cutaneous ligaments should be released at the level of retinacula cutis (Fig. 13-35, 36), and usually the anteromedial cheek should be augmented.

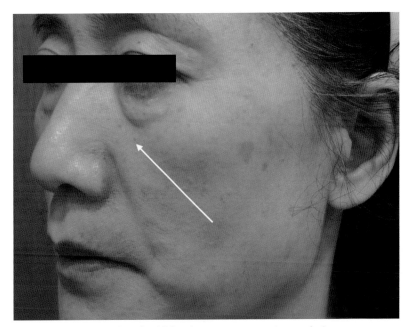

Fig. 13-35 **Nasojugal and midcheek groove correction technique**

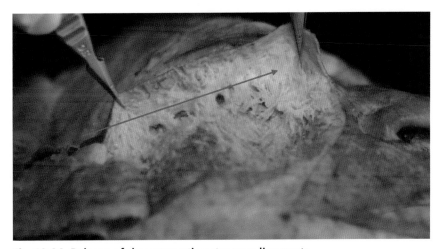

Fig. 13-36 **Release of the zygomatic cutaneous ligaments**

A 23G blunt-tip microcannula is moved back and forth at the retinacula cutis level, and moderate resistance and tearing of the fibrous tissue would be felt. When the cannula movement changes to weaker resistance after approximately ten back-and-forth movements, start to inject filler.

It is recommended to pinch the borderline of the groove by the non-injecting hand because of restriction of filler migration.

13. 2. 2. 3. 2 Filler amount

When inject just midcheek groove, 0.5~1 mL/side is needed, and when inject anteromedial cheek together, 1~2 mL/side would be injected.

13. 2. 2. 3. 3 Progress and photograph

A case of corrected midcheek groove and anteromedial cheek together: 2 mL of filler is injected unilaterally (Fig. 13-37).

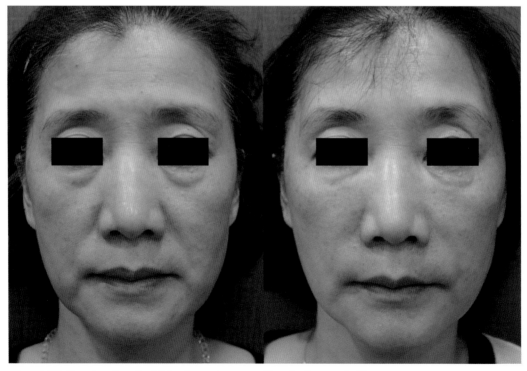

Fig. 13-37 **Nasojugal and midcheek groove correction: before and after**

13. 2. 2. 3. 4 Cautions

Midcheek groove would worsen without enough release of zygomatic cutaneous ligaments.

Among the Oriental people, 30% have infraorbital trunk (detoured branch) of the facial artery at the subcutaneous level (Fig. 13-38). Palpation of arterial pulsation before injection would be helpful in preventing vascular compromise.

It is essential to move gently to release the zygomatic cutaneous ligament to minimize damage of adjacent tissues.

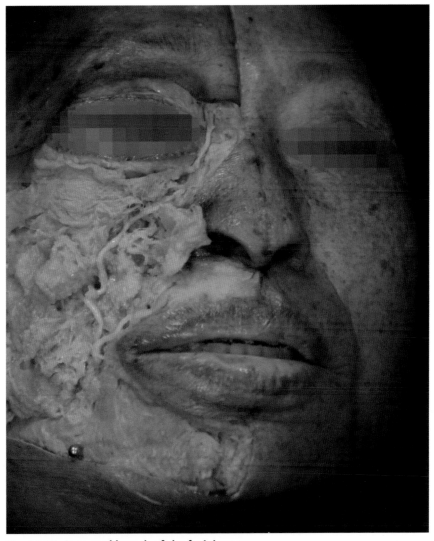

Fig. 13-38 **Detoured branch of the facial artery**

Suggestive Readings

1. Wong CH, Hsieh MK, Mendelson B. The tear trough ligament: anatomical basis for the tear trough deformity. Plastic and reconstructive surgery. 2012;129(6):1392-402.
2. Alghoul M, Codner MA. Retaining ligaments of the face: review of anatomy and clinical applications. Aesthetic surgery journal. 2013;33(6):769-82.
3. Mendelson BC. Anatomic study of the retaining ligaments of the face and applications for facial rejuvenation. Aesthetic plastic surgery. 2013;37(3):513-5.
4. Rossell-Perry P, Paredes-Leandro P. Anatomic study of the retaining ligaments of the face and applications for facial rejuvenation. Aesthetic plastic surgery. 2013;37(3):504-12.
5. Wong CH, Mendelson B. Facial soft-tissue spaces and retaining ligaments of the midcheek: defining the premaxillary space. Plastic and reconstructive surgery. 2013;132(1):49-56.
6. Pessa JE, Rohrich RJ. Facial topography: clinical anatomy of the face: CRC Press; 2014.
7. Yang HM, Lee JG, Hu KS, Gil YC, Choi YJ, Lee HK, et al. New anatomical insights on the course and branching patterns of the facial artery: clinical implications of injectable treatments to the nasolabial fold and nasojugal groove. Plastic and reconstructive surgery. 2014;133(5):1077-82.
8. Wong CH, Mendelson B. Midcheek Lift Using Facial Soft-Tissue Spaces of the Midcheek. Plastic and reconstructive surgery. 2015;136(6):1155-65.
9. Kim H-J, Seo KK, Lee H-K, Kim J. Clinical Anatomy of the Face for Filler and Botulinum Toxin Injection: Springer; 2016.

Infraorbital groove and hollowness

Gi-Woong Hong, M.D., Ph.D., Plastic Surgeon

13. 3. 1 Definitions

A groove in the infraorbital region (GIR) refers to a narrow furrow around the infraorbital rim, and hollowness of the infraorbital region (HIR) refers to a sunken space in the infraorbital area. They can develop together or separately in the aging process. Either the groove or hollowness needs correction because it causes a fatigue appearance. However, whether it is creased or sunken, it is called a tear trough. However, since the procedure should be performed according to the causes, it is important to provide a definition and classification. In the Oriental people, it is rare that the orbital bone is depressed and the skin and soft tissues are relatively thicker than those in Western people, so indentation along the orbital rim borderline would just appear. Infraorbital groove can be divided into the tear trough deformity on the medial side and orbitomalar groove on the lateral side. The osteocutaneous retaining ligament is usually found at the site between the thin skin of the eyelid portion and thick skin of the nasal and anteromedial cheek portion. Among them, tear trough deformity is located at the medial 1/3 depressed area of the lower eyelid, inferomedial to the orbit, and its length is less than 3cm. It is a natural depressive crease from the medial canthus to the vertical line of medial pupillary line and could be seen in some young people for anatomical reasons. Usually in the aging process, the groove deepens and connects to the palpebromalar groove, finally presenting as a long crease.

Nasojugal groove is located in the medial part of midcheek groove and sometimes confused with a tear trough, but they have different causes and shape and should be differentiated by anatomy. Tear trough develops between the palpebral and orbital portions of the OOM, but nasojugal groove formats between the medial orbital portion of the OOM and origin of levator labii superioris alaeque nasi (LLSAN) muscle. The medial part of the OOM orbital portion becomes narrow and inserts to the medial canthal tendon. Thus, the tear trough, which is located above the band, and nasojugal groove, which is located below the band, tend to fuse at the medial canthal area. The nasojugal groove develops when the medial band of the OOM orbital portion is strong and through contraction of the LLSAN muscle, and it is shallower than the tear trough. The nasojugal groove is almost at the same location medially but runs lower than the tear trough laterally. When the nasojugal groove is severe, it tends to connect to the midcheek groove by zygomatic cutaneous ligament, and all these creases are called united groove (Fig. 13-39).

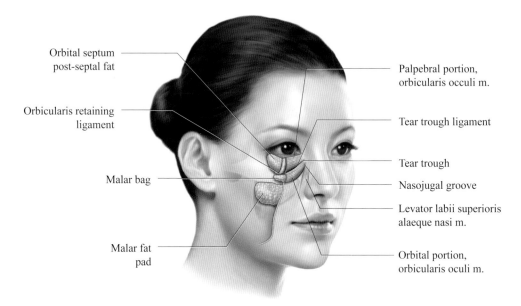

Fig. 13-39 DDx between the tear trough and nasojugal groove

Infraorbital hollowness can be divided into three classes as follows:

- Class 1: Medial orbit area depression accompanies the tear trough and minimal flattening of the central cheek area.

- Class 2: Since the medial part of the orbital depression deepens, tear trough and nasojugal groove develop together, and usually the lateral part of the orbit is also depressed. It is accompanied with anteromedial cheek mild volume deficiency and mild flattening of the central cheek triangle.

274

• Class 3: Circumferential depression along the orbital rim. The palpebromalar groove or lid-cheek junction groove is seen laterally. Anteromedial cheek depression and also reverse triangle of the central cheek can be seen. Thus, the nasojugal groove deepens, connects with the oblique midcheek groove, and is accompanied with malar bag. In Western people, when there is infraorbital hollowness, the palpebral portion of the OOM also changes into a deeper and thinner skin, but in Oriental people, this part appears bulged because of orbital fat bulging.

13. 3. 2 Anatomical considerations

As described previously, tear trough is located between the palpebral and orbital portions and in the cephalic border of the malar fat pad and attaches a few millimeters below the orbital rim. There were theories that the medial part of the OOM tends to attach to the bone and lateral part of the orbicularis retaining ligament is attached to the ligamentous muscle. However, recent anatomical literatures reveal that the medial part also has a TTL that pulls the skin as the lateral part.

There are various causes of infraorbital groove. In the TTL medially and orbital retaining ligament laterally, differences in skin thickness and texture of the lid cheek junction area and thickness of the subcutaneous fat layer and orbital fat bulging aggravate the groove.

When there is a strong medial muscular band and LLSAN and LLS constrict, the nasojugal groove tends to be prominent. Moreover, the groove tends to deepen when attached to the midcheek groove.

Infraorbital hollowness has more developed symptoms as described above, and the SOOF under the arcus marginalis decreases in volume. The TTL, which is the true osteocutaneous ligament, originates from the maxillary bone to the skin and is located between palpebral and orbital parts of the OOM. It starts from the medial canthal tendon insertion level just below the anterior lacrimal crest and elongates to the medial pupillary line laterally. From this point, it connects to the orbicularis retaining ligament, which is composed of upper and lower lamella, and these two ligaments extend to the lateral orbital thickening at the level of lateral canthus. The medial part of the orbicularis retaining ligament is tighter than the lateral part, so lateral hooding tends to occur. The lateral part is relatively easy to inject with a filler because releasing the ligament is easier and there are also loose spaces below the OOM.

The TTL has a similar structure with the zygomatic cutaneous ligament histologically. The TTL can be seen more prominently by tethering effect when frowning. To fill this area, it is recommended to inject beneath the ligament and push it superficially. Otherwise, the filler would migrate above the ligament and deepen the groove.

In the aging process, tear trough deformity would deepen due to loss of skin elasticity, orbital fat protrusion, orbital bone and soft tissue absorption, and midface ptosis. Thus, an additional procedure might be needed to solve other presenting problems (Fig. 13-40).

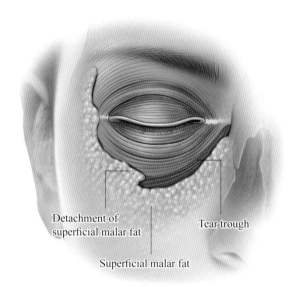

- Tear trough deformity is located from the medial canthus to the cheek area and natural ptosis in the aging process.
- Patient in the early 20s can also have tear trough deformity due to anatomical differences.
- Tear trough deformity might be prominent because of adjacent tissue volume loss.
- Aging process: prominent eyelid bags, loss of periorbital fat, and loss of skin elasticity

Detachment of superficial malar fat

Tear trough

Superficial malar fat

Fig. 13-40 Infraorbital changes combined with tear trough deformity

A midcheek groove or furrow is seen at the zygomatic cutaneous ligament, from the upper medial side to the lower lateral side. Moreover, this ligament is attached from the periosteum to skin and divides into the upper and lower parts of the superficial and deep malar fat pads. DMCF is located below this ligament and, in the aging process, loses volume, and superficial fat pads such as nasolabial fat and medial cheek fat should fall downward because of lack of supporting structures. However, superficial and deep fat pads including the SOOF above the zygomatic cutaneous ligament do not migrate to downward in the aging process because the ligaments are supporting tightly, so when making facial expression such as a smile, the ligament holds the skin tightly by fibrous band and aggravates the midcheek groove. Patients tend to demand just midcheek groove or combined problems such as in the anteromedial cheek area. Midcheek groove tends to extend to the nasojugal groove by one continuous or disconnected line. The zygomatic cutaneous ligament is usually located at the point of disconnection (Fig. 13-41).

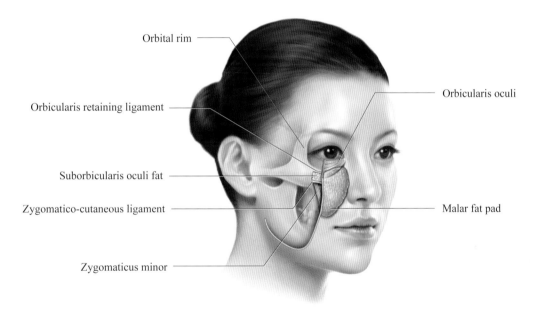

Orbital rim

Orbicularis oculi

Orbicularis retaining ligament

Suborbicularis oculi fat

Zygomatico-cutaneous ligament

Malar fat pad

Zygomaticus minor

Fig. 13-41 **Zygomatic cutaneous ligament**

The angular vein is located at the submuscular layer along with the nasojugal groove. The duplex facial artery infraorbital branch is seen in 30% of Oriental people and runs medial the inferior orbit and lower eyelids. This vessel runs between the SOOF and lower border of the lateral part of the deep medial cheek and runs upward at the medial border of the OOM, so care should be taken on the pathway. Moreover, the medial branch of the infraorbital artery runs along the nasojugal groove and superficially at the level of the fused area of the nasojugal groove and tear trough, so care should be taken.

13. 3. 3 Technique

From the anterior lacrimal crest to medial orbit, the OOM attaches to the bone tightly without any superficial or deep fatty tissue. In other tear trough areas except this part, there are superficial and deep malar fats. The deep fat layer underneath the muscle is called the SOOF, and there are medial and lateral SOOFs. The medial SOOF is located from the medial limbus line to vertical line of the lateral canthus, and the lateral SOOF is located from the vertical line of the lateral canthus to the borderline of temporal fat pad (usually horizontal line of the lateral canthus). The medial part of the tear trough consists of tight band, and there is no layer like the SOOF, so it is almost impossible to inject below the muscle. Thus, when injecting the filler, inject into or onto the muscle. Injection of a soft filler should be

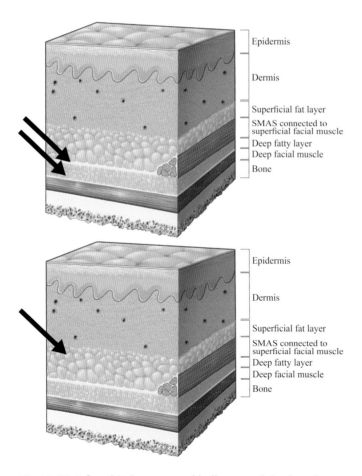

Epidermis

Dermis

Superficial fat layer
SMAS connected to
superficial facial muscle
Deep fatty layer
Deep facial muscle
Bone

Epidermis

Dermis

Superficial fat layer
SMAS connected to
superficial facial muscle
Deep fatty layer
Deep facial muscle
Bone

Injection plane

- Submuscular or supraperiosteal, except for the area near the medial canthus

  1) Submuscular injection of HA filler at the lid/cheek junction area (including the SOOF, palpebromalar groove, and middle and lateral orbital areas)

  2) Tear trough area – interspace or upper space of muscular origin of the OOM because the submuscular space is very tight, and there is no SOOF in the medial portion

  3) Subdermal injection of HA filler at the medial end because thinning of skin is severe due to deficiency of subcutaneous tissue volume and to smooth out other irregular surfaces.

Fig. 13-42 **Infraorbital groove and hollowness: injection plane**

performed near the muscle at the tear trough and lateral part of the SOOF, and if there is any irregularity, it is recommend to inject a very soft filler at the subdermal layer (Fig. 13-42).

Multiple veins including the inferior palpebral vein are located at the infraorbital area, and when there is mild sunken or only depressed medial tear trough, it is better to inject using a needle, but care should be taken on the veins. However, when it is depressed widely, it is recommended to use a cannula. The infraorbital nerve and artery perforate the infraorbital foramen 8~10 mm below the orbital margin and vertical line of the medial pupillary line. Thus, the entry point would be 15~20 mm below the orbital margin and vertical line from the lateral limbus, and this point could also avoid the zygomaticofacial nerve and artery, which are located lateral to this point (Fig. 13-43).

Insert the cannula and gently place the cannula tip at the desired area. Use the fanning technique in the depressed region and retrograde linear threading technique in the groove (Fig. 13-44).

As described previously, the medial part of the tear trough does not have subcutaneous tissue. It is recommended to inject a very soft filler at the subdermal layer to correct the crease. Moreover, when there is any irregularity, inject a soft filler at the subdermal layer additionally (Fig. 13-45).

Injection entry point and direction

1) It is 1.5~2 cm apart from the lower orbital rim margin on the vertical midline of the lateral limbus for infraorbital hollowness only.
2) The lateral part of midcheek (1.5~2 cm apart from the lower orbital rim margin) on the vertical line of the lateral orbital rim inner margin for infraorbital and midcheek hollowness

- Toward the tear trough and palpebromalar groove under the muscle, including the SOOF, except for the medial portion – intramuscular injection for the medial portion of the tear trough

Injection technique

- Retrograde fanning and linear threading injection
- Very slow release

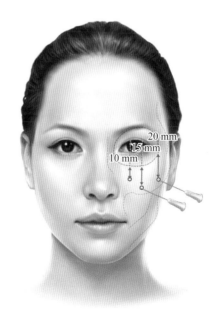

Fig. 13-43 Infraorbital groove and hollowness: injection point

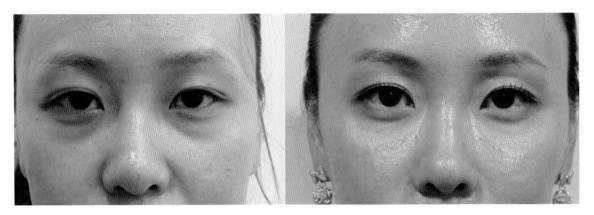

Fig. 13-44 Infraorbital groove: before and after

Injection entry point and level

- For the medial end of tear trough deformity and other irregularly depressed portions after deep injection
- Subdermal injection to augment the fine depressed medial portion of the tear trough deformity and to smooth out the surface around the rim

Injection technique

- Droplet technique all around the rim under the dermis
- Tenting technique for fine depressed medial end
- Vital Light or diluted Restylane Vital 0.2~0.3 mL for each area: 33G nanoneedle

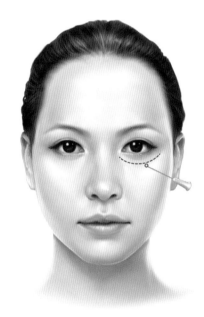

Fig. 13-45 Infraorbital groove and hollowness: needle injection technique

The nasojugal groove is located between the medial and lateral parts of the DMCF and SOOF, so to avoid vessels described previously, make an entry point on the lateral side of this area.

To correct midcheek groove, a cannula should be used to release the lateral fibrous band; the entry point would be the vertical line from the lateral orbital rim and horizontal line from the alar groove (Fig. 13-46).

Midcheek groove injection entry point

- Lateral portion of the groove requiring volume
- Lower portion of the midcheek groove around the vertical line of the lateral orbital rim and horizontal line of mid-alar groove

Mid-cheek groove injection technique

- Linear threading and layering technique after undermining, if required
- Perlane or SubQ 0.7~1 mL for each area of the midcheek groove: 27G needle or 23G cannula
- Restylane Lidocaine 0.3~0.5 mL for each area for subdermal injection to smooth out the surface

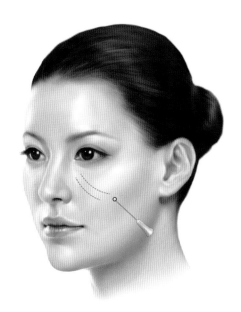

Fig. 13-46 Midcheek groove: injection point and techniques for cannula

To correct midcheek groove, the fibrous band should be undermined beneath the groove using 21~23G cannula. Sufficient release should be performed to make a space for the filler; otherwise, a more depressed groove might be observed. After release, inject the filler at the deep malar fat pad including SOOF by retrograde linear threading and layering technique. Moreover, injection at the superficial malar pad can be performed if required, and subdermal injection might be needed at the fibrous band area. It is recommended to check the result by moving of face such as smiling, if there is any lump or dislocation of the filler.

In the correction of the infraorbital groove or hollowness except midcheek groove, it is recommended to design at the sitting position and make an entry point. When injecting using a needle, care should be taken regarding the veins. For an accurate injection, the patient should open the eyes. Gentle injection, to prevent lumps, and gentle massage after injection are recommended. Moreover, orbital fat should not be penetrated. The infraorbital area tends to swell, so cooling pack application for 24 h is suggested. Do not try to perform perfect injection at once, but try undercorrection, and additional injection is recommended after 2 weeks (Table 13-1).

Table 13-1 Injection procedure for infraorbital groove and hollowness

Do:
1. Have the patient sit up for the injection, with a fixation on the opened eye
2. Avoid vascular structures
3. Inject under the OOM (except for the medial canthus)
4. Undercorrect
5. Gently mold or sculpt after injection to avoid irregularities
6. Inject slowly so as not to create a bolus under the skin
7. Inject in 2 sessions 2~4 weeks apart. Undercorrect 70% at first session and 30% at second session
8. Stay below the infraorbital fat pad
9. Use caution around the lacrimal and lower eyelid fat pad
10. Instruct the patient to apply cooling pack over the treated area in the next 24 h to reduce edema and ecchymosis, if required
Do not:
Inject more than 0.5 mL on each side per session

Inject filler at the infraorbital groove or hollowness. Bruising, swelling, tenderness, and hematoma are likely to develop, and the Tyndall effect or irregular beading might develop when injecting superficially. Thus, overcorrection at once should not be performed, and usually 0.3~0.5 mL is injected at once (Table 13-2).

Table 13-2 Side effects of HA filler injection for infraorbital groove and hollowness

(1) Bruising
(2) Swelling
(3) Tenderness
(4) Hematoma
(5) Visible irregularities (beading) : especially when injecting superficially
(6) Overcorrection
(7) Accentuation of mid-cheek groove : due to change of subcutaneous fat or dermal component
(8) Visible gel (Tyndall effect)

The effectiveness would decrease in the following conditions, so additional procedure should be considered carefully: severe skin laxity, very thin skin, severe pigmentation, prominent orbital fat, severe allergy or swelling, previous low blepharoplasty history, and other scars.

Suggestive Readings

1. Yang HM, Lee JG, Hu KS, et al. New anatomical insights on the course and branching patterns of the facial artery: Clinical implications of injectable treatments to the nasolabial fold and nasojugal groove. PlastReconstr Surg. 2014;133:1077-1082.

2. Koh KS, Kim HJ, Oh CS, Chung IH. Branching patterns and symmetry of the course of the facial artery in Koreans. Int J oral Maxillofac Surg. 2003;32:414-418.

3. Stutman RL, Codner MA. Tear trough deformity: review of anatomy and treatment options. Aesthetic Surgery Journal, 32(4):426, 2012.

4. Wong CH, Hsieh MK, Mendelson B, The tear trough ligament: Anatomical basis for the tear trough deformity. PlastReconstr Surg. 129:1392, 2012.

5. Mendelson BC, Muzaffar AR, Adams WP, et al. Surgical anatomy of the midcheek and malar mounds. PlastReconstr Surg. 110:885, 2002.

13-4 Infraorbital groove and hollowness

Yong-Woo Lee, MD, MBA, Plastic Surgeon

13. 4. 1 Design (Fig. 13-47, 48)

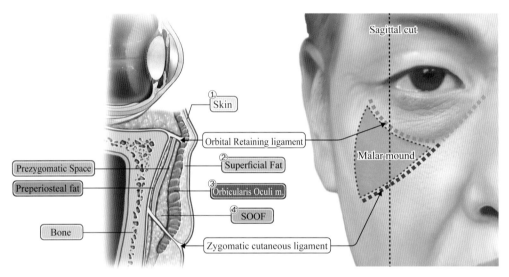

Fig. 13-47 **Anatomical borderlines of infraorbital groove and hollowness, Sagittal view at the palpebromalar and midcheek groove**

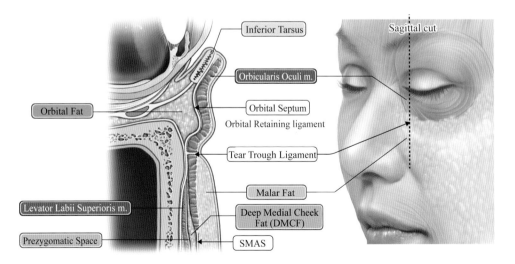

Fig. 13-48 **Sagittal view at the tear trough deformity**

13. 4. 2 Anesthesia

Local lidocaine injection at the entry point is performed.

13. 4. 3 Technique

13. 4. 3. 1 Needle versus cannula

Puncture through the lateral part of the entry point, and inject at once including the medial part using 23G 3.2 cm needle.

13. 4. 3. 2 Filler amount

Less than 0.5 mL/side is used. When addition amount is needed, it is recommended to inject after 2 weeks.

13. 4. 3. 3 Cautions

When correcting the tear trough deformity and orbitomalar groove, always consider the orbicularis retaining ligament. It is the true osteocutaneous ligament. The TTL tends to pull skin harder than the orbitomalar groove, so tear trough deformity is more difficult to correct. When there is abrupt angle groove, superficial injection might be needed but may result in lump formation, so only a small amount should be injected. Furthermore, the Tyndall effect would occur when the skin is thin.

In contrast, the orbitomalar groove has a relatively loose connection, so subcutaneous injection can provide good results. Tear trough deformity and orbitomalar groove should be corrected by injection of filler at the lower part of the ligaments.

Midcheek groove, which is called Indian band, is located lateral to the midpupillary line and at the zygomatic cutaneous retaining ligament. This portion also pulls the skin tightly, so deep and subcutaneous injection is needed. This area has relatively thick skin, so Tyndall effect usually does not occur but should be considered. Moreover, lump formation should be considered when making facial expression. When there is infraorbital hollowness combined with anteromedial cheek depression, volume augmentation in a wide area might be needed. Fatty tissue changes and aging process are wide and extensive processes. Correction of the groove could result in an unharmonious appearance, so anatomical aging process should be known.

13. 4. 3. 4 Complications and management

There are many vessels located in this region, and bruising might occur when the vein is ruptured. The angular vein tends to run on the lateral end of the tear trough, so it might be ruptured. To avoid this vein, inject at reverse Trendelenburg position, and local anesthesia including epinephrine or any vaso-constriction method might be helpful. Sitting position is also helpful to estimate filler amount.

The infraorbital nerve perforates the infraorbital foramen and is located in this area. When filler injection is performed deeply, care should be taken regarding this nerve, and it is recommended to avoid injection when the patient complains of severe pain or feeling resistance at the cannula tip.

The infraorbital area is less related to ocular complications because the medial end of the tear trough is the only place to meet the angular artery. However, since there is a detoured facial artery, compression of the medial canthal portion might prevent the complication.

Suggestive Readings

1. Huang YL, Chang SL, Ma L, Lee MC, Hu S. Clinical analysis and classification of dark eye circle. International journal of derma-tology. 2014;53(2):164-70.
2. Wong CH, Hsieh MK, Mendelson B. The tear trough ligament: anatomical basis for the tear trough deformity. Plastic and recon-structive surgery. 2012;129(6):1392-402.
3. Stutman RL, Codner MA. Tear trough deformity: review of anatomy and treatment options. Aesthetic surgery journal. 2012;32(4):426-40.
4. Haddock NT, Saadeh PB, Boutros S, Thorne CH. The tear trough and lid/cheek junction: anatomy and implications for surgical cor-rection. Plastic and reconstructive surgery. 2009;123(4):1332-40; discussion 41-2.
5. Lambros V. Observations on periorbital and midface aging. Plastic and reconstructive surgery. 2007;120(5):1367-76; discussion 77.

Infraorbital groove and hollowness correction at a glance

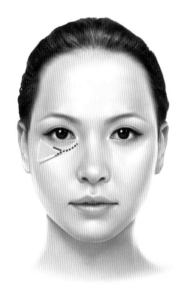

- Dr. Choon-Shik Youn (Dermatologist)'s technique

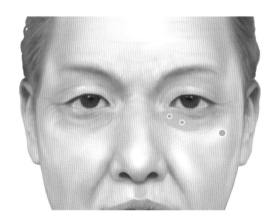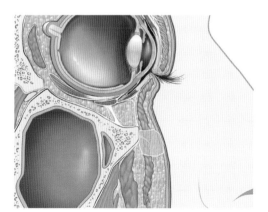

- Dr. Hyun-Jo Kim (Dermatologist)'s technique

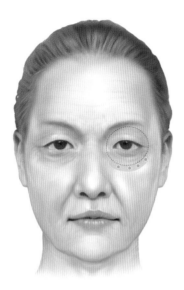

• **Dr. Gi-Woong Hong (Plastic Surgeon)'s technique**

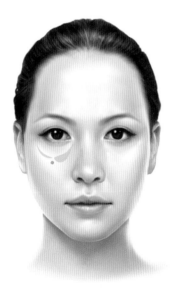

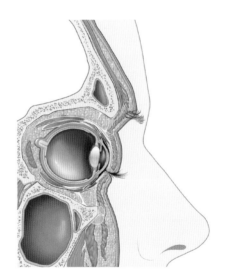

• **Dr. Yong-Woo Lee (Plastic Surgeon)'s technique**

	Dr. Youn (Derma)	Dr. Kim (Derma)	Dr. Hong (PS)	Dr. Lee (PS)
Needle/cannula	30G	23G cannula and/or 33G needle	30G cannula 30G needle	23G needle
Unilateral amount	0.4~0.8 mL	0.2~0.4 mL	Deep: 0.3~0.5 mL Superficial: 0.2~0.3 mL	Approximately 1 mL
Elasticity The Chaeum	No.1 or 2	No. 1 or 2	No. 1	No. 2
Anesthesia	EMLA cream application	EMLA cream application/regional nerve block	Cannula: entry point lidocaine injection Needle: EMLA cream application	Local lidocaine injection
Techniques	Linear threading technique	Linear threading and bolus injection technique	Retrograde fanning and linear threading for deep injection Microdroplet and tenting for superficial injection	Bolus
Layer	Tear trough: into muscle or submuscular Palpebromalar groove: SOOF	Periosteum and/or subcutaneous layer	Deep: 1) Middle and lateral orbit: SOOF under the OOM 2) Medial orbit: intermuscular space Superficial: subdermal	SOOF if possible periosteum

Pretarsal fullness

14-1 Pretarsal fullness

Gi-Woong Hong, M.D., Ph.D., Plastic Surgeon

14. 1. 1 Considerations before injection

The lower eyelid margin where the tarsal plate is located has a 2 mm width, and the inner side is concave in shape and well attached to the eyeball, and outer side is roll in shape and called pretarsal fullness. The OOM tarsal portion is located in front of the tarsal plate, and when smiling, it looks like rolled cake above the subtarsal line. Oriental people like to have pretarsal fullness because the face looks cute and young and the eye appears bigger. Excessive fullness would make the eyes smaller, so adequate fullness is needed. Obtaining pretarsal fullness in young people is for a pretty appearance. However, because of the aging process, skin laxity, OOM atrophy, and drooping occur, and this results in loss of pretarsal fullness. The patient shows a fatigue and monotonous appearance, so pretarsal fullness is needed. Moreover, skin darkness and fine wrinkles might also improve (Table 14-1).

Table 14-1 Effects of pretarsal fullness: bulkiness and contraction of OOM

- Large eye effect
- Pretty and young appearance
- Improved dark circle
- Fine wrinkle removal (by skin expansion)
- Three-dimensional effect of infraorbital area

When designing, let the patient smile and draw the subtarsal line. Never inject under the line, and usually, it is 5~6 mm below the subciliary line. The shape would be evenly distributed from the medial to lateral canthus or thick lateral portion. To obtain thick lateral pretarsal fullness, it is better to make the lateral 1/3 thickest. Thus, the shape would be different by patient's preferences, and injection could be performed using a needle or cannula, but a needle is recommended for a more precise shape.

14. 1. 2 Technique

When using a needle, inject directly at the desired point. When using a cannula, make an entry point few millimeters lateral to the lateral canthus and augment the lateral to medial part by retrograde small volume injection technique, linear threading technique, and serial puncture and tenting technique gently and slowly (Fig. 14-1).

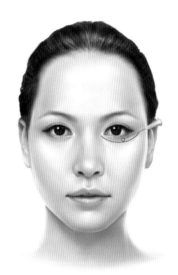

Injection technique

- Linear threading
- Retrograde tiny injection
- Very slow release
- Serial puncture and tenting

Fig. 14-1 **Pretarsal fullness: injection technique**

If we use a hard filler, it is likely to be irregular in shape and has excessive protrusion, so a soft filler should be used. When injected too deep, it is likely to result in swelling as a whole and not pretty bulging shape, and if injected too superficial, it is likely to show irregular shape, partial protrusion, and Tyndall effect. The author likes to inject into the OOM and subdermal layer to obtain an overall shape and then at the subdermal layer for smooth contour (Fig. 14-2).

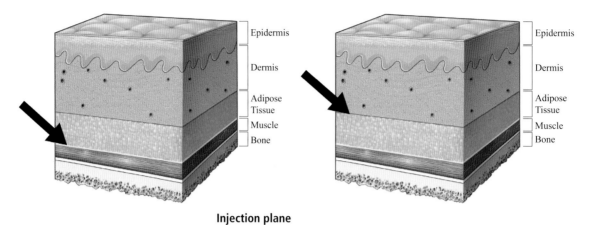

Injection plane

- Deep subdermal injection
- Subdermal injection for even surface
- Close to eyelash

Fig. 14-2 **Pretarsal fullness: injection plane**

The filler should be injected as close as possible to eyelash, and orbital fat bulging should be considered because sometimes pretarsal fullness and orbital fat bulging might fuse and looks swollen when the patient smiles.

Pretarsal fullness injection is not recommended in certain cases, which are lack of preexisting eyelid roll muscles, too narrow or wide eye fissure, too high or low lateral canthus, severe enopthalmos or exophthalmos, very thick skin, very dark color skin, severe skin laxity, excessive septal fat bulging, and previous low blepharoplasty scar (Table 14-2).

Table 14-2 **Contraindications of pretarsal fullness**

- Absence of muscle for eyelid roll formation
- Too wide or narrow eye fissure
- Too high or low eye slant
- Deep set or protruding eyes
- Too thick lower eyelid skin
- Severe infraorbital dark circle
- Lower eyelid scar due to previous surgery
- Severe skin laxity
- Excessive lower eyelid orbital fat bulging

Among these, people with previous lower blepharoplasty status usually have flat pretarsal area, so it is better to obtain pretarsal fullness, but few things should be considered. In case of ectropion due to scar, it is better not to perform injection. In case of not severe scar, it is recommended to inject not deeply initially because the filler would not be injected at the scar but below it. Therefore, it is recommended to inject superficially at the initial and deeper place. Because of scar adhesion, it would show irregularity, but when the eyelids open and close for 1 or 2 weeks, the filler would be distributed evenly. When irregularity still exists after a time, inject the filler at the depressed area using a microneedle.

Suggestive Readings

1. Chen MC, Ma H, Liao WC. Anthropometry of pretarsal fullness and eyelids in oriental women. Aesthetic plastic surgery. 2013;37(3):617-24.
2. Putterman AM. Facial anatomy of the eyelids. Plastic and reconstructive surgery. 2004;113(6):1871-2; author reply 2-3.

14-2 Pretarsal fullness

Yong-Woo Lee, M.D., M.B.A., Plastic Surgeon

14. 2. 1 Design

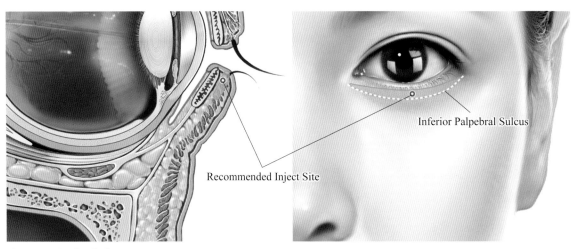

Recommended Inject Site

Inferior Palpebral Sulcus

Fig. 14-3 Sagittal view

14. 2. 2 Anesthesia

Lidocaine injection at the entry point is performed.

14. 2. 3 Technique

14. 2. 3. 1 Needle versus cannula

The author prefers to inject from the lateral entry point and from medial to lateral part using a 25G needle. Additional injection is performed using a 29~31G needle.

14. 2. 3. 2 Filler amount

Approximately 0.5 mL/side is used. Additional injection should be considered because hyaluronic acid filler tends to pull adjacent water, so undercorrection is considered at initial injection.

14. 2. 3. 3 Cautions

Inject as close to the eyelash as possible. There is too much resistance when injecting near the eyelash after all, so the filler would be injected in loose areas. Most unsatisfactory results are obtained when the filler is located under the desired place. Since there is an eyeball behind and the area could not be massaged after injection, it is important to inject evenly the first time. Use two cotton swabs, one on the conjunctival side and another on the skin side, to push injected filler to the upper side. It is not necessary to inject by touching the tarsus. There is a very small amount of fat between the tarsus and OOM, so filler injection into the muscle is recommended. It is more effective to obtain pretarsal fullness when injecting into the subcutaneous layer, but usually the lower eyelid skin is very thin and would lead to a Tyndall effect.

14. 2. 3. 4 Complications and management

The most common complication is ruptured vessel. Once the vessel ruptures, bulging immediately appears, and it is difficult to inject the filler evenly. Therefore, we recommend injecting after swelling subsides. These area vessels have a small diameter like the supraorbital area, so embolism might not occur.

Suggestive Readings

1. Chen MC, Ma H, Liao WC. Anthropometry of pretarsal fullness and eyelids in oriental women. Aesthetic plastic surgery. 2013;37(3):617-24.
2. Liew S, Nguyen DQ. Nonsurgical volumetric upper periorbital rejuvenation: a plastic surgeon's perspective. Aesthetic plastic surgery. 2011;35(3):319-25.
3. Kim YK, Kim JW. Evaluation of subciliary incision used in blowout fracture treatment: pretarsal flattening after lower eyelid surgery. Plastic and reconstructive surgery. 2010;125(5):1479-84.

14-3 Pretarsal fullness

Hyun-Jo Kim, M.D., M.S., Dermatologist

14. 3. 1. Design

Usually pretarsal fullness is made by upper superficial fat constriction when the OOM palpebral part constricts. It could be seen in almost everyone when smiling, but the degree is variable.

When there is prominent pretarsal fullness in the unexpressed face, it is a very unnatural appearance. It could be made natural looking by injecting as close to the eyelid margin as possible (Fig. 14-4).

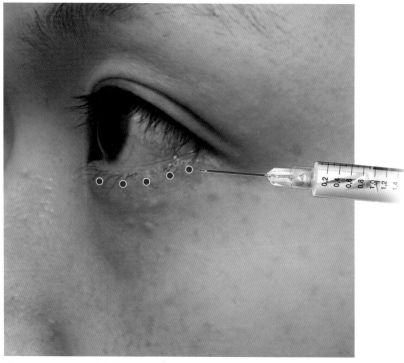

Fig. 14-4 **Pretarsal fullness augmentation**

14. 3. 2 Anesthesia

EMLA cream application is sufficient, and the filler containing lidocaine could be injected without any anesthesia.

14. 3. 3 Technique

14. 3. 3. 1 Needle versus blunt-tip microcannula

Both can be used. The author prefers to inject 3~5 points using 33G needle because a small amount of filler is needed.

14. 3. 3. 2 Filler amount

A small amount is sufficient: 0.1~0.2 mL/side could lead to satisfactory results.

14. 3. 3. 3 Progress and photograph

In a case with an injected amount of 0.2 mL/side, natural pretarsal fullness is observed when smiling (Fig. 14-5, 6).

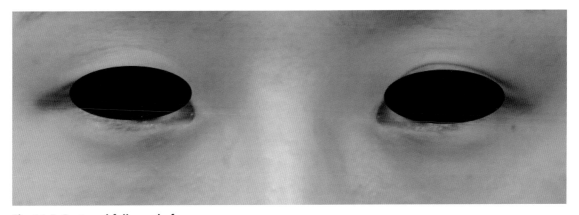

Fig. 14-5 **Pretarsal fullness: before**

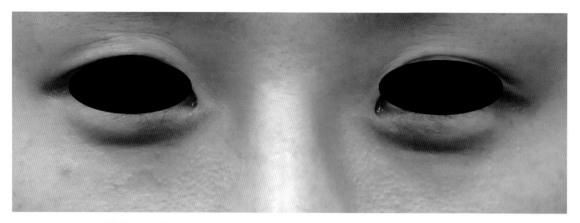

Fig. 14-6 **Pretarsal fullness: after**

14. 3. 3. 4 Cautions

Inferior palpebral artery arcades run behind the OOM, so it is recommended to inject at subcutaneous fat level to prevent vascular compromise (Fig. 14-7).

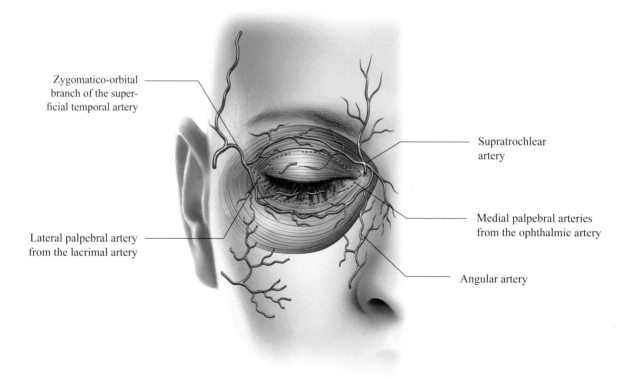

Zygomatico-orbital branch of the superficial temporal artery

Supratrochlear artery

Lateral palpebral artery from the lacrimal artery

Medial palpebral arteries from the ophthalmic artery

Angular artery

Fig. 14-7 **Dangerous arteries in pretarsal fullness augmentation**

Suggestive Readings

1. Kim H-J, Seo KK, Lee H-K, Kim J. Clinical Anatomy of the Face for Filler and Botulinum Toxin Injection: Springer; 2016.
2. Han J, Kwon ST, Kim SW, Jeong EC. Medial and lateral canthal reconstruction with an orbicularis oculi myocutaneous island flap. Archives of plastic surgery. 2015;42(1):40-5.

Pretarsal fullness augmentation at a glance

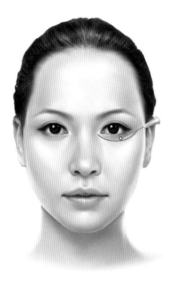

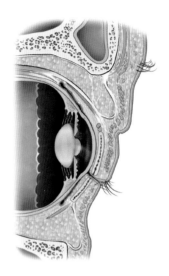

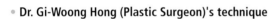

- Dr. Gi-Woong Hong (Plastic Surgeon)'s technique

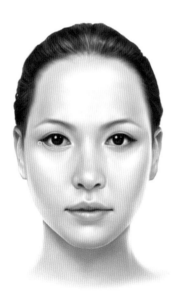

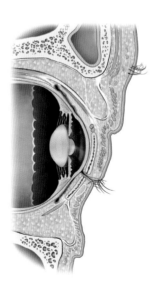

- Dr. Yong-Woo Lee (Plastic Surgeon)'s technique

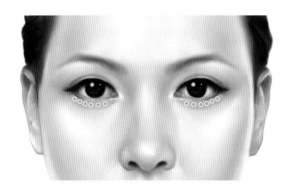
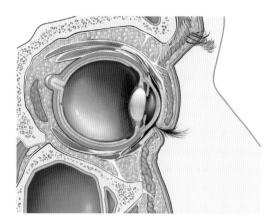

• **Dr. Hyun-Jo Kim (Dermatologist)'s technique**

	Dr. Hong (PS)	Dr. Lee (PS)	Dr. Kim (Derma)
Needle/cannula	Cannula 30G Needle 30G	Needle 25G, 1.25in	Needle 33G
Unilateral amount	0.2~0.3 mL	0.1~0.2 mL	0.1~0.2 mL
Elasticity The Chaeum	No. 1	No. 2	No. 1
Anesthesia	Cannula: lidocaine injection at the entry point Needle: EMLA cream application	Local lidocaine injection	EMLA cream application
Techniques	Cannula: Retrograde small volume injection with linear threading technique Needle: Linear threading with serial puncture technique	Bolus technique	Bolus (point) injection
Layer	Inject at the upper muscular space for volumization and superficial subdermal space tenting	As close to eyelash as possible Inject close to the tarsus	Subdermal or subcutaneous layer

Index

CERTIFICATE OF
ENGLISH EDITING

This document certifies that the paper listed below has been edited to ensure that the language is clear and free of errors. The edit was performed by professional editors at Editage, a division of Cactus Communications. The intent of the author's message was not altered in any way during the editing process. The quality of the edit has been guaranteed, with the assumption that our suggested changes have been accepted and have not been further altered without the knowledge of our editors.

TITLE OF THE PAPER

Practical guidelines for effective and safe filler injections: Filler techniques based on anatomical deliberation by 13 experts

AUTHORS

Lee Won

JOB CODE

CHEIL_50

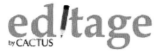

Signature

Vikas Narang

Vikas Narang,
Vice President, Author Services, Editage

Date of Issue
August 25, 2018

Editage, a brand of Cactus Communications, offers professional English language editing and publication support services to authors engaged in over 500 areas of research. Through its community of experienced editors, which includes doctors, engineers, published scientists, and researchers with peer review experience, Editage has successfully helped authors get published in internationally reputed journals. Authors who work with Editage are guaranteed excellent language quality and timely delivery.

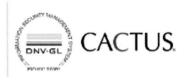

Contact Editage

Worldwide	Japan	Korea	China	Brazil	Taiwan
request@editage.com	submissions@editage.com	submit-korea@editage.com	fabiao@editage.cn	contato@editage.com	submitjobs@editage.com
+1 877-334-8243	+81 03-6868-3348	1544-9241	400-005-6055	0800-892-20-97	02 2657 0306
www.editage.com	www.editage.jp	www.editage.co.kr	www.editage.cn	www.editage.com.br	www.editage.com.tw